Social Media for Medical Professionals

David R. Stukus • Michael D. Patrick
Kathryn E. Nuss

Social Media for Medical Professionals

Strategies for Successfully Engaging in an Online World

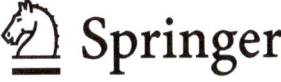 Springer

David R. Stukus
Nationwide Children's Hospital and The
Ohio State University College of Medicine
Columbus, OH
USA

Michael D. Patrick
Nationwide Children's Hospital and The
Ohio State University College of Medicine
Columbus, OH
USA

Kathryn E. Nuss
Nationwide Children's Hospital and The
Ohio State University College of Medicine
Columbus, OH
USA

ISBN 978-3-030-14438-8   ISBN 978-3-030-14439-5   (eBook)
https://doi.org/10.1007/978-3-030-14439-5

This Springer imprint is published by the registered company Springer Nature Switzerland AG.
The registered company address is: Gewerbestrasse 11, 6330 Cham, Switzerland

Foreword

When I started my campaign of medical advocacy on social media, I walked uphill waist deep in snow both ways.

Okay, maybe not quite. But that is what it felt like.

The reality is there were very few doctors online publicly and most who were seemed less interested in medical facts and more invested in foods that bust belly fat.

Sigh.

Back then, medical societies also told doctors that being on social media was unprofessional. All of these early guidelines seemed written by people, mostly older men, who had never been on social media in any meaningful way. A bit like me, a gynecologist, trying to tell an orthopedic surgeon about operating on the ankle.

Eye roll.

But I didn't care what anyone said because I knew social media was where my patients were. And getting accurate information to people matters, especially as most of us are prone to believing the first piece of data that we collect. I also knew that at one point in time, we doctors felt the telephone was terribly unprofessional, and yet, here we are with excellent telephone triage guidelines for many medical conditions.

Almost 16 years ago, my family experienced a medical catastrophe. I was pregnant with triplets, and one of my sons died at birth, and my other two sons were born extremely prematurely. They were very ill for a very long time – and like everyone else, I turned to the Internet for medical information. What I found was almost impossible to navigate. And I began to wonder: If I am a doctor and I am falling down snake oil-infested rabbit holes, how does everyone else manage?

I decided when my kids were a little better that I was going to try to fix the medical Internet. I know, a pretty naive goal. However, I am sure, at one point, people thought surviving at 26 weeks – the age my children were born – was impossible, and yet here I am with two amazing young men who fill my life with joy.

It is hard for people to wade through the quagmire that is the medical Internet. Bad information is everywhere, fear sells, and the lure of the cure is so potent. In our 24/7 news cycle, a misleading medical story can not only do damage itself but can also spawn tens and sometimes even hundreds of other erroneous headlines resulting in millions of impressions. Sometimes, the articles are even accurate, but the headlines are terribly misleading. Let's face it, many of us, doctors included, don't always read to the end of a story.

We all mistake repetition for accuracy, a phenomenon called the illusory truth effect. And social media, with easy retweets and reposts, is the very model of repetition.

The glut of medical misinformation is real. And medical professionals who are invested in accuracy and helping patients must help. The biggest barrier that I hear about engaging online is that it looks so hard and seems so complicated! How does one even get started?

That is why *Social Media for Medical Professionals* is such an important book. Trying to understand the myths that may be holding you back from engaging, what avatar to use, how and when to engage, what content works and what doesn't, and knowing the risks (there are a few, like all medical interventions)—all this and more is presented for you in a clear and concise manner. I wish this book had been around back when I said to myself, "Gunter, you should try this Twitter thing out and see what happens!"

Sometimes I wonder if social media were around when Andrew Wakefield presented his fraudulent data to the world if an army of medical professionals could have taken to social media to shut him down and expose him within weeks? Maybe people wouldn't be dying from measles right now? Maybe all of that money we spent proving over and over again that vaccines are safe and don't cause autism could have been used to find an effective therapy or a cure for another condition?

Interesting thoughts.

Social media is already affecting the medical care you deliver to your patients. But it is also affecting you medically on a personal level. Medical misinformation on social media is affecting the fluoride in your drinking water. It is exposing you and your family unnecessarily to vaccine-preventable illnesses. It is telling lies about reproductive health that affects how people vote.

Not engaging doesn't seem to be an option. Everyone deserves access to quality and accurate health information, and medical professionals are uniquely poised to help. Dr. David Stukus and his coauthors have given you the blueprint you need to get started, so you can help make the medical Internet better for everyone.

I look forward to seeing you online!

Dr. Jen Gunter
@DrJenGunter a.k.a. Twitter's resident gynecologist

Preface

If you're tired of seeing false medical claims flood your inbox, actors or actresses using their celebrity status to rave about unproven medical treatments, or trying to convince patients (or friends and family members) why they should follow the evidence-based treatment plan discussed with their physician and not spend money on those fancy energy crystals they saw on Instagram, then this book is for you. The Internet and social media have created an incredible means to connect with people from across the world in real time. Unfortunately, these avenues can also be exploited for evil through rampant misinformation, fake news, and creating a culture where patients trust the anonymous members of their Facebook group more than their personal doctor.

The three of us each have different clinical interests and backgrounds but found one another due to our shared interests and experiences in using social media to help our patients. Collectively, we have led workshops at national medical conferences, have given talks to audiences of various backgrounds, and have developed and incorporated curriculum for an elective rotation at our institution that trains medical students and residents about social media. The reason we wrote this book was to lend our experience and approach to all of you – medical professionals with various backgrounds, interests, and audiences. After all, we are all in this together.

Each chapter in our textbook will discuss unique aspects regarding social media and how it pertains to medical professionals. Whether you're a physician, a nurse, or a pharmacist, we offer tools and strategies that you can start utilizing today in your online pursuits. Our book covers a range of topics and strategies that are useful regardless if you don't know your hashtags from your retweets, or if you're a seasoned social media veteran with thousands of followers.

Feel free to skip around on your journey. Some sections of our book may not pertain to your interests at this time, or some of you may not be ready for the higher-level strategies we discuss. This book was written in a manner that allows each chapter to stand alone or can be read straight through in order. Undoubtedly, some of the platforms we discuss will be obsolete in the near future. That is why we took a purposeful approach to provide a broader discussion and practical tips that will stand the test of time and can be utilized whether you're using Facebook, Twitter, YouTube, or whatever fun new channel yet to be invented.

We feel the time has come to reclaim our role as trusted medical professionals. It's time to help patients and the public understand the differences between pseudoscience and trusted information. It's time to fight back against those who deliberately misinform patients with false claims of miracle cures in the name of profit. If you've read this far, that means you're with us and we are so glad to have you on board. Thank you for taking the time to read our book – we hope it provides a blueprint and ideas for how you can help grow and educate a broader audience.

Please feel free to reach out to any of us through social media – you know where to find us.

Columbus, OH, USA   David R. Stukus, MD
                                                                          Michael D. Patrick, MD
                                                                          Kathryn E. Nuss, MD

Contents

1 Social Media: Changing the Human Experience 1
David R. Stukus
What Is Social Media? 1
Out with the Old 2
Leave a Message: LOL 3
Social Media Platforms 4
It's Gone Viral! 5
My Example 5
Bots and the Rise of Fake News 8
Social Networks 10
Facebook 10
    Facebook for Healthcare Professionals 12
YouTube 12
    YouTube for Healthcare Professionals 14
Instagram 14
    Instagram for Healthcare Professionals 15
Twitter 16
    Twitter for Healthcare Professionals 18
Reddit, Snapchat, Pinterest…The List Goes On and On 18
LinkedIn and Doximity 20
Conclusion 21
References 21

2 A Brief History of Digital Communications 23
Michael D. Patrick
In the Beginning… 23
Compu-Serv 25
Usenet and Newsgroups 25
Network Growth 27
The Internet and World Wide Web 28
Advanced Browsers and the Rise of Websites 29

America Online.   31
Physicians Online   32
Broadband Connections   33
Search Engines   35
Advanced Web Programming Languages.   36
Blogs.   37
RSS Feeds.   38
Podcasts.   38
Social Networking Sites   39
Smartphones and Mobile Apps.   42
Conclusion   44
References.   44

3   **Myths That Prevent Medical Professionals from Engaging**   49
Michael D. Patrick
Myth 1: People Use Websites, Not Social Media, to Find
Answers Related to Health and Wellness   49
Myth 2: Millennials Are the Only Generation Using Social Media.   50
Myth 3: Healthcare Consumers Don't Need My Help.   52
Myth 4: I'm Not Changing Anyone's Mind   53
Myth 5: I'm Too Old (or Not Techy Enough) for Social Media.   54
Myth 6: Social Media Involvement Takes Too Much Time   55
Myth 7: Large Audiences Are Required to Make a Difference   55
Myth 8: Comments Are My Own; They Do Not Represent
My Employer   57
Myth 9: Social Media Engagement Is Too Risky   58
Myth 10: My Patients Won't Leave Me Alone   59
Myth 11: I Don't Get Anything in Return.   60
Myth 12: Other Providers Already Participate in
Social Media… I'm Not Needed   61
Conclusion   62
References.   62

4   **The Role of Medical Professionals in Social Media**   65
David R. Stukus
A Common Scenario.   65
The Power of Anecdotes   66
The Quality of Evidence Matters   70
The Echo Chamber Effect.   73
Cognitive Bias.   74
Heuristics   76
Pseudoscience 101   77
Why Healthcare Professionals NEED to Be Engaged in Social Media . .   80
I'm a Doctor on Social Media, but I'm Not YOUR Doctor   81
Conclusion   82
References.   82

5   The Art of Digital Storytelling 83
Michael D. Patrick
Why We Should Become Storytellers. 83
Introducing the Reporter Questions 85
What Do We Want People to Know? 86
Why Do We Want Them to Know?. 87
Who Do We Want to Tell?. 88
How Can We Best Tell Them? 90
It's Story Time!. 91
    When Is the Best Time to Tell Our Story? 92
    Where Is the Best Place to Tell Our Story? 93
    Engage the Audience. 94
    Curate Great Content 95
    Create Great Content. 96
    Putting It All together 97
Conclusion 100
References. 100

6   If You Tweet It, They Will Come 101
David R. Stukus
Start with Your Profile. 101
Consider Your Audience Before Yourself 104
Think Like a Patient 107
Twitter 101: How to Engage 110
Take Advantage of Trending Topics 111
Hashtags 114
Time Management 116
Use Metrics to Increase Engagement 117
Conclusions. 120
References. 120

7   Content Curation 121
Kathryn E. Nuss
Social Media as a Pipeline to Knowledge. 122
Finding Credible Sources About Healthcare on the Internet
Can Be Difficult 124
What It Means to Be Credible 125
Credibility Red Flags 126
This is Why It's Essential for Healthcare Professionals
to be Smart Online!. 127
How Using Social Media Can Help Healthcare Professionals 128
How Social Media Helps Patients. 129
Who Are You Online?. 130
Amazing Role Models 131
    Step by Step Pediatrics 132
    Wendy Sue Swanson MD 134

     Dr. Kevin Pho   136
     Dr. Dave Stukus @AllergyKidsDoc   137
     Dr. Eric Topol   138
   Examples of Excellent Content.   139
   Amazing Content Ideas.   140
   Conclusion   142
   References.   142

8   **Content Creation**.   145
   Kathryn E. Nuss
   Building an Assortment of Unique Content   145
   Why Original Content?.   146
     The SEO Factor.   146
   Sometimes You Have to Create Your Own Content   147
     Administrative Organization and Social Media   147
     Local Health Concerns   148
   Developing a Content Plan   148
   Your Content Creation Depends on Who Your Audience Is   149
   Creating a Content Calendar.   149
   Platforms for Excellent Content Creation.   151
     A Website!.   151
     Blog Posts   151
     Facebook.   153
     Twitter.   154
     LinkedIn   154
     YouTube   154
     Podcast Platforms   155
     Instagram.   156
   Examples of Good Content Creation   157
     Pull Together Studies as Quick Posts   157
     Curate Screenshots to Illustrate Content.   157
     Pull Together the Latest News   157
     Curate Content Published by Top Sites in Your Niche   157
     Post Powerful Quotes   158
     Make Your Own GIFs or Share Your Favorite GIFs   158
     Reference the Pamphlets from Your Own Office   158
     Record a Quick Video Educating About a Common Health
     Concern, Frequently Asked Health Questions, etc.   158
     Patient Testimonials   158
     Podcasts.   158
     Create your Own Infographics   159
     Exploit Trendy Topics.   159
     Organize Contests.   160
     Use High-Quality Stock Photography   160
   Cross-Promoting on Social Media   160
     Cross-Posting Is Not Cross-Promoting.   160

Useful Tools 161
  Hashtagify.me 161
  SlideShare and SlideSnack 161
  Grammarly 162
  Giphy 162
  Vidyard 162
  SurveyMonkey 162
  Anchor 162
  Typeform 163
  Typorama 163
  Animoto 163
  Placeit 163
  Canva 163
  Hootsuite 163
Role Models of Content Creation 164
  Dr. Howard Luks 164
  Dr. Sandra Lee (aka Dr. Pimple Popper) 164
  New York Dynamic Neuromuscular Rehabilitation 164
  Dr. Wendy Sue Swanson (Seattle Mama Doc) 164
Be Careful! A Word of Caution 165
The Difference Between Good and Great Content 166
See How You're Doing: Analyzing Social Media Statistics 168
  Page Views 168
  Organic Likes and Traffic 168
  Conversion Rates 168
  Engagement Rates 169
  Audience Growth 169
  Demographic Metrics 169
  Google Analytics 169
  Sprout Social 169
Conclusion 170
References 170

9 Dos and Don'ts: Social Media Tips for the Medical Professional 173
Diane Davis Lang
Social Media Policy 173
Confidentiality 174
Disclosing Intellectual Property, Fair Use, and Creative Commons 176
Photos and Videos 179
Threats and False Statements 179
Harassment or Defamation 180
Explicit Content 180
Endorsements 181
Conducting Business on Social Media 182
Media Relations 182
Speaking on Behalf of the Organization 183

Complaint Protocol..   183
Crisis Communication   184
Maintain Appropriate Professional Boundaries   185
Organizational Reputation   186
Conclusion   186
References..   186

10   How to Spot and Deal with Internet Trolls........................ 189
Callista M. Dammann
How to Deal with Trolls: Strategies for Dealing with Negative
Comments and Feedback   189
Types of Trolls   190
     The Grammar and Spelling Troll   190
     The Political Troll..   190
     The Insult Troll...   192
     The Bad Experience Troll...................................   192
     The Topic Trolls (Also Known as the Persistent Debate Troll)   193
     Extremist Troll   195
Tips for Dealing with Trolls   196
     So, Why Do People Become Social Media Trolls?
     (And How Not to Turn into One)   197
How to Have a Healthy and Productive Debate Online   198
Conclusion   201
References..   202

11   The Sky Is the Limit 203
David R. Stukus
Social Media and the Ivory Tower   203
Public Health..   205
Research   206
ZDoggMD..   210
Conclusion   212
References..   213

Index...215

Social Media: Changing the Human Experience

1

David R. Stukus

> *Toto, I've a feeling we're not in Kansas anymore*
>
> —Dorothy, Wizard of Oz

What Is Social Media?

Do you remember what it was like to take a roll of film to get developed? Have you ever returned from a dream vacation to learn weeks later that not only did your pictures get overexposed but also that "perfect picture" included a wayward thumb? Was your first mobile phone a flip phone? Do you have a Hotmail account? If you answered yes to any of these questions, then you likely remember what life was like before social media. Some would say that was a much simpler time when people relied on actual conversation and human interaction in order to communicate. Others wonder how relationships could exist without instant access to updates from everyone's lives. Whether you've adopted social media and have taken advantage of its many platforms, or you've led the resistance for the past decade…love it or hate it, social media is here to stay.

Broadly defined, social media refers to interactive computer-mediated technologies that facilitate the creation and sharing of information [1]. This can take various forms, including opinions, pictures, videos, or long-form written communication. In addition, social media involves the use of networks where individuals and communities can communicate with one another in real time and allow for exchange of ideas and commentary. While different social media platforms exist, they all share common features:

- *Interactive applications* – The Internet allows for rapid connection between anyone with a computer or smartphone.
- *User-generated content* – Each social media account, whether it represents an individual, a company, or an organization, can post their own content and comments. This sharing of ideas is the central element to social media.
- *Profiles* – Each account can establish a unique profile that serves as a representation of that person, organization, or group. The user profile serves as an

© Springer Nature Switzerland AG 2019
D. R. Stukus et al., *Social Media for Medical Professionals*,
https://doi.org/10.1007/978-3-030-14439-5_1

introduction to the world and allows other users to quickly identify whether they are interested in that user's content.

- *Social networks* – Social media platforms facilitate the connection of like-minded and similar accounts with one another by connecting a user's profile with other individuals or groups.

Out with the Old

Traditional media, such as magazines, newspapers, and television broadcasting, serves as a one-way forum to disseminate information. While content delivered in this manner may provoke verbal comments or elicit an emotional response, the consumer is unable to share their opinion with the content originator in real time. That dynamic changed with the advent of social media. Data from Pew Research in 2016 showed that 86% of Americans use the Internet and among those users, 80% use Facebook, 32% use Instagram, and 24% use Twitter [2]. Unlike previous unilateral dissemination of information, we can now communicate with one another in real time by leaving comments, asking questions, or offering opinions surrounding the content disseminated by others through social media. This is a substantial shift in the dynamic of how we each receive, interpret, and process information. In many ways, this elevates the information being shared by making it more interactive, personal, immediate, and intimate. Unfortunately, the ability to rapidly post comments or replies has removed the natural editing capabilities that occur when taking time to offer a thoughtful and measured response. Instead, emotional elephants often dominate the conversation.

As recently as 10 years ago, many of us received our political, scientific, or world news solely through reading newspapers or watching the evening news. By natural extension of the editorial process and production timeline, the information shared in this manner originated during the previous day or days, was limited in scope, and was subject to biases of the reporting agency. Today, if an important news story breaks, social media and websites afford instant access to multiple sources of information and opinions, including video, written description, and commentary. The way Americans receive their news has also changed, with 62% receiving it from social media [3]. Today, news cycles occur in a matter of minutes, not days, and reading the newspaper in many ways reflects a long-form reporting of "old" news that occurred days or weeks beforehand.

This paradigm shift has many benefits, as well as unintended consequences. Previously, reporters were afforded more time to cultivate stories, gather essential facts, and could wait until they had a more complete understanding of the subject matter before disseminating their findings. Today, media outlets are racing one another to provide the fastest reporting, which often does not allow for dissemination of complete or necessarily accurate information. Likewise, consumers are more apt to form rapid opinions based upon how the information is presented and their own internal biases…and can now share those opinions with the entire world within a matter of seconds. In addition, we are all too familiar with the knee-jerk claims of "fake news" by politicians and pundits when information counters their narrative or agenda. All of these factors have fundamentally changed how information is disseminated and obtained throughout the world.

Leave a Message: LOL

This dramatic shift in how we all receive and share information has resulted in changes in how we communicate with one another. Instead of taking the time to call someone on the telephone to have a conversation, the majority of people, particularly younger generations, prefer to use text messaging to communicate. Smartphone users in the United States send and receive five times as many texts compared with the number of phone calls each day, which averages about 26 minutes a day spent texting [4]. This is certainly much faster and efficient, but also makes it easier for ideas to be poorly communicated and misunderstood. Teenagers, in particular, can become withdrawn, have higher levels of stress, or feel socially isolated if they are not receiving a constant stream of text messages from their friends [5]. Regardless of whether someone is busy actually experiencing life through social engagements or travel, they are now expected to instantly share their story on any number of social media accounts. A catastrophic unintended consequence of the ubiquitous nature of smartphones and desire to capture photos of every human experience involves deaths that occur while taking selfies [6]. A study published in 2018 identified 259 deaths between October 2011 and November 2017 that occurred, while people were attempting to take selfies while visiting dangerous locations, partaking in risky activities, or deliberately ignoring warning signs. These findings were so alarming that the authors declared a need to post signs stating "No selfie zones" at tourist areas located near bodies of water, mountain peaks, and tall buildings.

Concerns about frequent social media usage and depression have been raised in recent years. An increasing number of research studies are attempting to

Table 1.1 Signs of social media addiction

Spending a lot of time thinking about social media or planning how to use it
  Preoccupation to share comments, photos, or thoughts immediately
  Over sharing of ideas, photos, and information
  Inability to judge appropriate nature of posts
Urge to use social media more and more over time
  Checking for updates to feed or responses during any downtime, regardless of how brief
  Leaving social media sites open on smartphone while engaging in other activities
Using social media to forget about personal problems
  Social media becomes a convenient escape and temporary relief from stress and problems
  Constant distraction from activities, takes longer to complete tasks
Becoming restless or troubled if prohibited from using social media
  Withdrawal symptoms can occur if cut off from social media sites, i.e., lack of cellular service
Overuse of social media has had a negative impact on relationships
  Become more comfortable engaging online than in person
  Replace time spent with friends/loved ones with social media groups
  Can lead to fear of face-to-face communication

characterize the prevalence of social media addiction, which occurs when online activities interfere with daily life, especially with functioning at work or school (Table 1.1). Online harassment, or "cyberbullying," is a real problem that can dramatically impact someone's mood and quality of life. Previously, if someone wished to insult or offend another person, they had to confront them face to face or at least leave a menacing voice mail message. Now, users can spew hatred and offensive language from behind a wall of anonymity on social media, but the intended consequences are very real and felt by the recipient. While the dark side of social media has received increased attention in recent years, there is currently little that can be done to prevent or eliminate these negative aspects.

Social Media Platforms

It is challenging to define the evolving social media services, but there is some agreement among experts regarding the distinct types of social media, which are highlighted in Table 1.2. In 2016, Merriam-Webster defined social media as "forms of

Table 1.2 Various types of social media

Platform	Features
Blogs	Online journal or informational website
	Allows longer format sharing of views
Business networks	Interaction with businesses or individuals with similar personal or career interests
Collaborative projects	Allows users to build communication, problem-solving, research, and critical thinking skills
	Exposes users to different viewpoints
Enterprise social networks	How a business or organization uses social media to connect with individuals or organizations who have shared interests
Forums	Message boards where people can hold conversations and post comments
Microblogs	Combination of blogging and instant messaging that allows users to create short messages for sharing with an online audience
Photo sharing	Uploading personal photographs to share with friends and family members
	Allows users to add photos and create a group album
Products/services review	Allows individuals who have purchased or used certain products or services to leave comments online regarding their experience
	Can help businesses reach larger audiences
Social bookmarking	A way for people to store, organize, search, and manage web pages
	Differs from bookmarks in a folder on a personal computer; this allows for access from any computer
Social gaming	Playing games online with groups of other players or users which encourages social interaction as opposed to playing games in solitude
Social networks	Dedicated application that allows users to communicate with each other, post information, leave comments, and send messages
Video sharing	Ability to share videos with a personal network, such as friends or family members
Virtual worlds	An online community environment designed and shared by individuals to interact in a custom-built simulated world

electronic communication (such as websites) through which people create online content communities to share information, ideas, personal messages, etc." Initial social media platforms included features such as instant messaging but have since expanded their reach and capabilities through incorporation of more engaging features.

Ultimately, social media is used to document and share memories, learn about new concepts, advertise oneself or business, form friendships, and grow ideas through content creation. Individuals can now build expansive networks in collaboration with other networks to help create and manage content.

It's Gone Viral!

Some social media platforms allow for rapid sharing of content to a large number of users. "Going viral" is a term that stems from viral infections, which spread rapidly from person to person. A social media post or site that goes viral is shared with large numbers of users very rapidly, which increases exposure of that account and can generate large numbers of new followers. Twitter's retweet option, Pinterest's pin function, and Facebook's share option all allow for rapid sharing and resharing of ideas to a large number of users.

My Example

I have had Twitter posts go viral on a few occasions, but my first experience is the most memorable. In 2014, the largest Ebola outbreak in history occurred in West Africa and garnered significant media attention [7]. Ebola first appeared in 1976 and epidemics have occurred sporadically over the past several decades. The epidemic in 2014 became the most widespread and deadly on record, resulting in more than 28,000 cases and over 11,000 deaths. Infection from Ebola causes rapid onset fever, severe headache, muscle pain, and weakness and kills almost half of individuals who become infected. Infection is spread very easily from contact with any infected person's bodily fluids. It often originates in underdeveloped parts of the world and can cause massive infection and deaths throughout a community. There is no cure for Ebola, and the only treatment is supportive care to try and keep someone alive as their organs fail and then hopefully recover. Given the rural nature of these outbreaks and limited healthcare in these low socioeconomic communities, many people do not receive effective treatment.

As horrific as an outbreak such as this can be for those living in remote parts of the world, attention and concern grew in 2014 when a few individuals with exposure on the front lines and/or acute symptoms traveled to the United States. Suddenly, Ebola was no longer a disease affecting people living in remote areas on a different continent, but it was now in the backyard of every American (or so the media made it seem). As discussed earlier in this chapter, in this instance, social media helped fuel rapid dissemination of information that was incomplete, incorrect, or created with the intent to garner a fear-based emotional response in the name of more website clicks.

During the same time frame, anti-vaccine sentiments were growing in increasing numbers among concerned parents. Vaccines have a long track record of safety and efficacy through use in millions of children and well conducted and numerous research studies. There is no debate regarding the dramatic reduction in serious infectious diseases such as polio, pertussis, rotavirus, and measles, among children across the world who have received vaccines. While anti-vaccine sentiments have been present since the origin of vaccine development in the late 1700s, social media has allowed a new platform for a well-organized and vocal anti-vaccine contingent to disseminate their views. In 2000, measles was declared eliminated from the United States. However, in recent years, as more and more parents have elected to not vaccinate their children due to unfounded concerns that vaccines cause autism or contain large amounts of toxic substances, measles outbreaks have occurred in various parts of the United States. Needless to say, the misinformation surrounding vaccines is rampant online and through social media, and this topic can generate an emotional response.

As a pediatric allergist and immunologist, I have received specialized training in regard to the immune system and am often asked to evaluate children with suspected immune deficiency. In the midst of the Ebola outbreak in 2014, one of my colleagues relayed a story of their interaction with a parent surrounding the influenza vaccine. I thought this was an interesting and timely commentary and formulated this tweet, shown in Fig. 1.1. At the time, I had approximately 1000 followers and was very careful to not violate any patient privacy laws or relay any identifiable information (see Chap. 9 for more information regarding the protection of patient privacy on social media).

I sent this out on a Wednesday morning, around 11 am EST. I checked my account around noon and noticed a few dozen retweets and several comments. By 3 pm, I received a notification from Twitter that my account, @AllergyKidsDoc was trending in Toronto. This meant that the algorithm used by Twitter at the time determined my profile was being mentioned, retweeted, or commented on more than

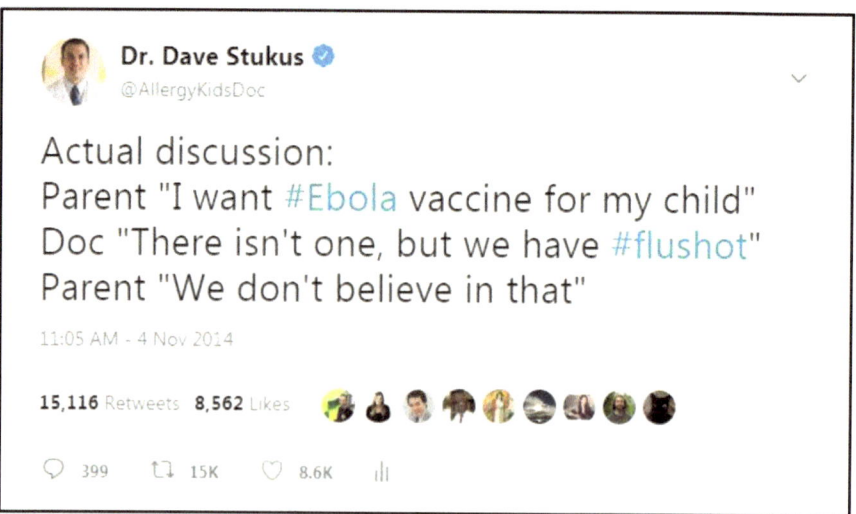

Fig. 1.1 My first viral tweet. (Adapted from https://twitter.com/AllergyKidsDoc)

almost all other accounts or hashtags in a specified time frame. Within the hour, my tweet had been retweeted or commented on over 1000 times. I then received notifications that I was trending in New York, followed by Washington DC, and ultimately, across the United States.

I suddenly became very nervous and actually starting sweating and feeling my heart race. I had no control over and little understanding of what was happening at the time. I was worried that my employer would be upset or that people would start posting negative comments toward me (yes, doctors get cyberbullied, too). After 48 hours, and over 10,000 retweets, things settled down. My number of followers almost doubled, and I was contacted by several media outlets to discuss Ebola, influenza, and vaccines. Ultimately, Forbes magazine named my tweet one of the Top 10 Healthcare Tweets of 2014.

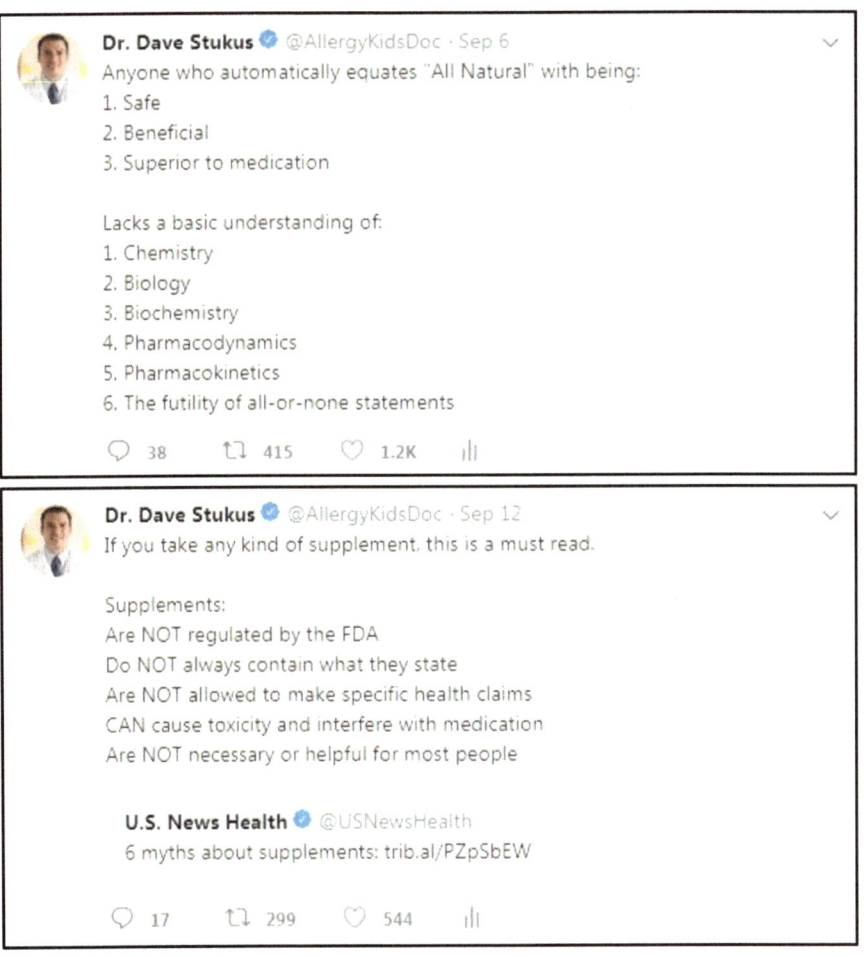

Fig. 1.2 Additional examples of viral tweets. (Adapted from https://twitter.com/AllergyKidsDoc)

Table 1.3 Elements of a viral tweet

Large number of followers	Having more followers allows for increased engagement and dissemination
	Increases the chance that a tweet will be noticed
Topic	Popular topics will gain more interest
	Trending topics will be noticed by more users at that particular time
Emotions	Tweets that garner an emotional response increase engagement; this can include laughter, crying, anger
Timing	Depends upon where most followers are located, i.e., a tweet sent at 3 am EST will have much less traction within the United States
	Tweets sent at the height of discussion surrounding trending topics will have the most engagement
Wording	Direct, clear, concise messages have the greatest impact
	No need to shorten words unless necessary
	Abbreviations used sparingly
Quality of attachment	High-quality, attention-grabbing pictures, videos, or GIFs will elicit more response
Links	Including a link to a reliable resource for additional information can increase dissemination
Hashtags	Use of the most popular or trending hashtags can increase how many followers read or retweet a post
Luck	The random nature of social media often plays a role in which tweets go viral or not. It often comes down to who is online at the time, who notices, and what their followers then notice

With experience, I have a better sense of why that particular tweet went viral and have since experimented with a similar approach to find less prolific, but similar, results (Fig. 1.2). My Ebola viral tweet included a popular hashtag, addressed two timely and emotional topics (Ebola and vaccines), and framed it in a way that relayed my observation from the viewpoint of a healthcare professional. In addition to thousands of accounts sharing that tweet with their own followers, there were hundreds of comments…and comments to the comments. This combination kept my Twitter handle as part of the overall impressions, which is what triggered the algorithm that determined I was trending. See Table 1.3 for additional elements that are common among viral tweets. I learned a valuable lesson as well: Always think before hitting send because once it's out there, it's out there.

Bots and the Rise of Fake News

An interesting phenomenon has accompanied the increased use of social media. Companies or individuals have developed ways to generate wide spread dissemination through the creation of bots. These are automated programs that can post content through multiple accounts and with great frequency, in a sense inundating users with their information and agenda. Chatbots and social bots are programmed in a manner that mimics natural human interactions. Their profiles often contain pictures of real people (frequently very attractive men or women, who may be scantily clad) and appear to be "human." The bot accounts then function in a manner similar to individual accounts and can like, comment, follow, or unfollow other users. At first glance, they are very difficult to tell apart from real people. However, careful

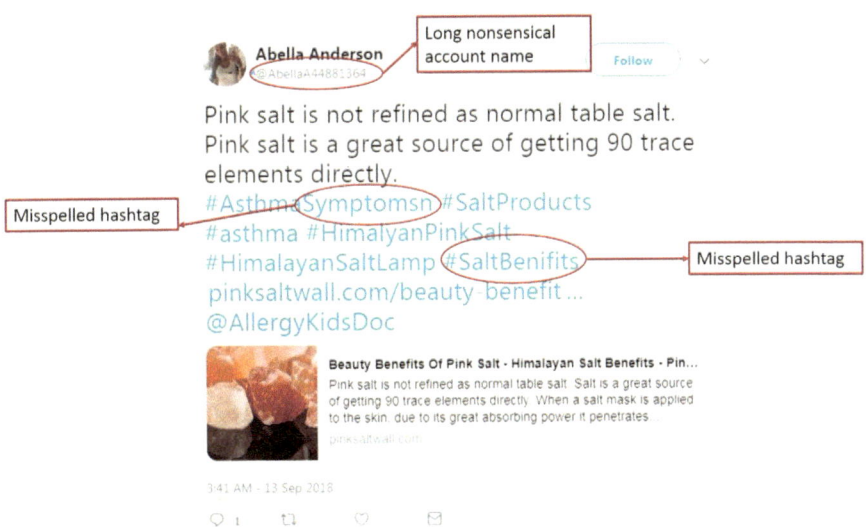

Fig. 1.3 Example of a bot promoting use of Himalayan salt. (Adapted from https://twitter.com/AbellaA44881364)

review of these accounts can reveal some features that make it less likely to be human in origin, including long account names that appear computer generated, misspelled words, and high volume of messages with little interaction. See Fig. 1.3 for one example of my encounter with a bot that generated a response directed at my account after I posted information surrounding Himalayan salts.

To make things more confusing, "cyborgs" are a combination of a human and a bot and are also used to spread fake news or create marketing buzz. Cyborgs can be bot-assisted humans or human-assisted bots. An example is a human who creates an account, sets automated posts and will interact from time to time with other users or comments. This allows the human to "cover their tracks" and prove that there is a real person behind the account, should it come into question.

These social bots, chatbots and cyborgs have made it difficult for companies to utilize data from their social media accounts to assist their marketing. Bots also have helped give rise to the rapid and pervasive dissemination of misinformation, particularly surrounding emotional topics such as vaccines, politics, and health-related information. Some of these bots have been traced to individuals or organizations that intend to influence voting strategies or purchasing habits among the general population or may be specifically targeted to social media accounts that have keywords or phrases in their profiles. Other bots seem to exist with the sole purpose of promoting chaos. Either way, every person who utilizes social media must now become savvy in regard to these bots or risk falling victim to their influence.

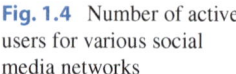

Fig. 1.4 Number of active users for various social media networks

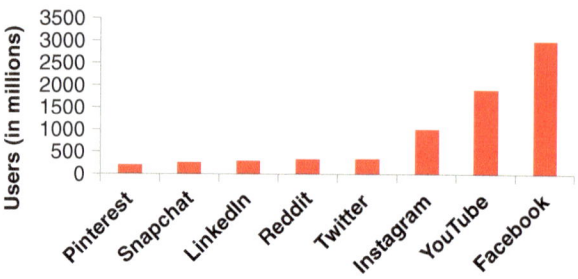

Social Networks

There are many networks people utilize, all of which share the central features discussed earlier, but differ in unique ways that attract different demographics. Figure 1.4 shows popular social networks according to number of active users in 2018 [8]. The following section will briefly discuss some of the most popular social networks but will not be all inclusive. Inevitably, given the rapid evolution of social media, some of these platforms may become obsolete in future years, and new ones will undoubtedly be developed.

Facebook

Initially launched in 2004, Facebook is the king of social media platforms. With over 2 billion active monthly users, Facebook was not only one of the earliest to arrive at the party, but its popularity has withstood both the test of time and competition from new social media sites. Each registered Facebook user can establish their own personal profile that reveals their posts and content. In 2011, the format of each user page was changed and became known as their "Timeline." The Timeline serves as a chronological feed of a user's stories, status updates, photos, interactions with other social media sites, and events. Users can add and edit at any time a larger photo/header at the top of their Timeline (Fig. 1.5).

The News Feed feature of Facebook appears on every user's home page and highlights information such as profile changes, upcoming events, and birthdays of the user's friends. The News Feed has been revamped over the past decade to remove unwanted features such as clutter or undesirable information and users can now control the type of information automatically shared with their Facebook friends.

Facebook connects users through the "friend" feature. Users can send requests for others to become their friend. Once accepted, friends can see all posts and information in the other user's Timeline. Users can also subscribe to a Facebook page, which allows access to that page's posts without becoming friends, i.e., posts from the account that does the subscribing will not show up in the Timeline of the account they have subscribed to – this is akin to one-way dissemination. The "like" button on Facebook was first enabled in 2009 and allows users to easily interact with status updates, comments, photos and videos, links, and advertisements. When the like button is clicked, that content appears in the News Feed of that user's friends and also displays the number of other users who liked the content. Instant messaging can occur through use of Facebook Messenger, which allows users to send

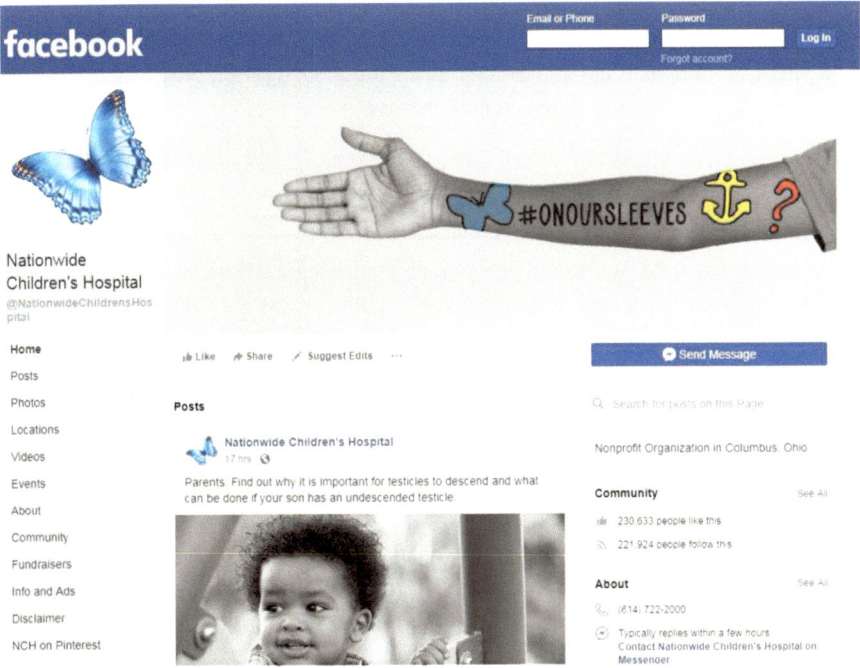

Fig. 1.5 Facebook home page for Nationwide Children's Hospital. (Adapted from https://www.facebook.com/NationwideChildrensHospital/)

messages to each other and chat without leaving the site. New features such as voice calls, video calls, and group conversations have been incorporated over recent years.

Facebook is used by individuals, businesses, organizations, and groups to provide information pertaining to the user's interests and also disseminate information from others. Privacy settings can be set to allow for sharing albums with only certain group members or for all Facebook users to have access. The "tag" feature allows users to label other Facebook users in the photo, which sends a notification to the friend that they have been tagged, along with a link to see the photo. In 2015, Facebook launched the "Instant Articles" program to provide articles from media and news organizations. This enables users to have access to articles without having to leave the Facebook site. This feature has been controversial as Facebook curators can suppress or promote news that supports various political agendas.

Facebook has significantly changed how families, friends, professional colleagues, and the world at large interact with one another. There are many positive aspects to this social media giant, including the ability to maintain a personal connection with friends, relatives, and acquaintances despite living long distances apart, to generate interest and income for businesses, and for rapid dissemination of information on a wide scale. However, Facebook has been subject to many criticisms and controversies over the past decade as well. Issues surrounding user's privacy, sharing user information with third-party trackers, facial recognition software, and its role in suppressing workplace and personal productivity are a few areas that have raised concern. Facebook has also received significant attention and criticism for providing a platform for conspiracy theorists, hate groups, and disruption of America's political process through dissemination of "fake news" and misinformation. Whether the impact has been good or bad, no one can dispute the enormous impact Facebook has had on the world.

Facebook for Healthcare Professionals

There are many ways healthcare professionals can use Facebook to disseminate information, interact with patients and the general public, grow their online presence, and promote their services. Facebook pages are essentially mandatory for any private practice, hospital, or professional organization that wishes to maintain relevance within search engines and be included when patients and consumers search online for health-related information. From an organization or practice standpoint, Facebook can be useful to relay information regarding hours of operation, location, professional services offered, as well as information regarding individual providers or any media related to the organization. These organizations can post links to articles, blog posts, and other content to help educate their patients and, as a by-product, attract new patients. Individual healthcare professionals can establish their own Facebook page for similar dissemination of information and to relay their professional affiliations, publications, and advocacy work. Facebook also provides an excellent platform for professional networking and connecting with colleagues from across the world.

YouTube

YouTube is a video sharing service launched in 2005 that allows users to watch, like, share, comment, and upload their own videos. YouTube is free to use and has served as a popular site for users to discover videos that match one's interests. If you can imagine a video, YouTube has it: music videos, comedy, how to guides, recipes, hacks, and more. Users can find clips from television shows and movies, video blogs, original videos, and educational videos. Both individual users and media corporations can upload videos and create their own channels, which allows for easy searching by other users. Motivated users can essentially create their own YouTube show and update content regularly, allowing them to disseminate information on a platform that most resembles traditional television viewing.

YouTube is now the second most popular social media site, with one billion hours of content being watched every day [9]. The popularity of YouTube stems from the video content, which is a visual method of sharing entertainment or information. Most videos are short, lasting only a few minutes, and are easily accessible across devices. YouTube allows videos to be embedded on any website through HTML but rarely allows downloading of videos. The quality of videos has increased over the past few years and is now available in high definition, which allows for pristine quality when viewing.

The face-to-face interaction that YouTube affords is appealing to users. This can enhance education through tutorials and demonstrations, lead to activism and grass roots political efforts, increase acquisition of news information, and increase access to government. For example, in 2007, the CNN/YouTube presidential debates allowed regular citizens to submit questions to United States presidential candidates via YouTube. Conversely, YouTube has allowed government officials to increase engagement with citizens, including the official White House YouTube channel.

A growing aspect of YouTube over recent years is the impact on young children. The developmental stages of children attract them to watching videos, which often contain their favorite cartoon characters or funny unexpected moments. YouTube videos often feature toys, popular characters they know, or people playing and having fun. Unexpected occurrences and odd events attract attention and interest as well. However, parents must be cautious as parody cartoon videos featuring popular characters behaving in mature and inappropriate manners have become popular viewing. Disturbing images of people being injured and sneaky advertising tactics are other areas to remain wary of as well.

As with other social media sites, there are potential negative aspects associated with YouTube. Despite its popularity among children, not all content is appropriate. Videos can be flagged if users find them inappropriate, and parents can also use the parental control feature to create a Safety mode and restrict access to mature videos. Cyberbullying can occur on this platform through the comments function on

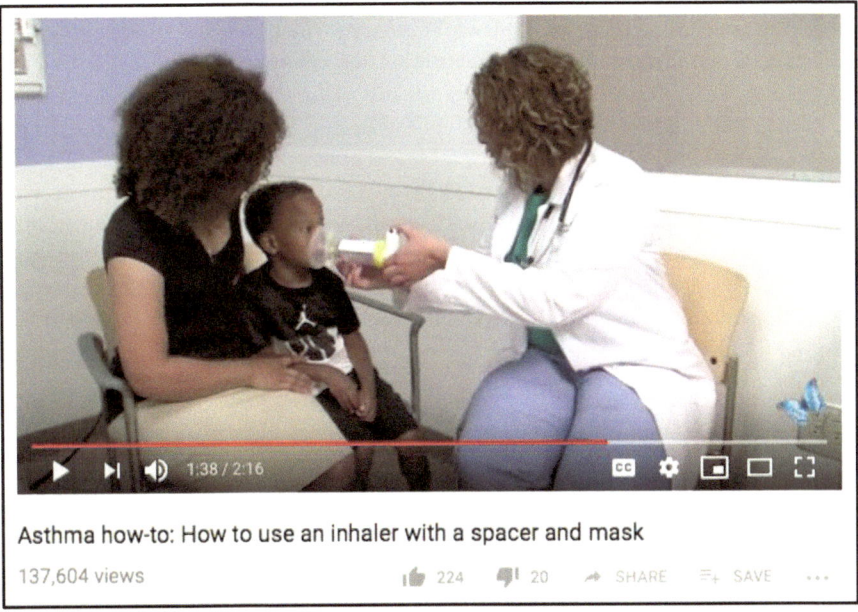

Fig. 1.6 YouTube video detailing the proper steps involved in administration of a metered-dose inhaler with holding chamber and face mask to a young child

YouTube. Users who upload videos can designate whether it is public, available for anyone to see, or private, available only through a direct link.

YouTube for Healthcare Professionals

YouTube is an interesting way for healthcare professionals to engage with a wide audience. Anyone can create and upload their own videos, which can be used to discuss evidence-based information pertaining to specific health conditions, demonstrate proper technique for medical devices (Fig. 1.6), or use cartoons or whiteboard videos to explain complicated health topics. Professional organizations and hospitals can use YouTube to create their own channels of video libraries that patients and the public can access. This can serve as an additional landing spot and enhance the online portfolio of professional practices, which can increase appeal for new patients, while also providing a service for existing patients. YouTube videos can then be shared across other social media platforms, allowing healthcare professionals to disseminate their creative educational content to a wider audience.

Instagram

Instagram is a photo and video sharing social network that is owned by Facebook. It launched in 2010 and, interestingly, is not centered on a website. Instead, users access Instagram through their mobile app, which is available across all mobile platforms, including iOS and Android. Photos and videos can be edited with various filters and organized with tags and location information. Accounts can be either private or public. Users can "like" photos or videos and follow other users to add their content to a feed. Instagram also allows users to create "Stories" with photos or videos that are only accessible for 24 hours after posting.

Instagram incorporates hashtags to help users search for common terms or words and locate content of interest. Instagram also has features to help users find content, including "Videos You Might Like" tab, an "Events" channel, and ability to search locations. A popular feature is the ability to apply filters to photos which can change the colors, contrast, tone, glow, and appearance. Users can also edit photos by adding text and drawings. Instagram users can interact with one another by leaving comments on posts, and conversations can occur by replying to the comments.

The allure of Instagram lies in the colorful and fun nature of sharing photos and videos. This allows for a personal peek into the user's life and has been a popular tool for celebrities to use to connect with their fans. Instagram has created careers for some users after they post photos or videos of themselves and created a genre of Instagram models, who gained their success purely as a result of the large number of followers they have on Instagram, which then created advertising revenue and other opportunities. A noted limitation of Instagram is that content curation and sharing is challenging as users cannot include links to articles or other sites through their posts. Users can creatively share information by incorporating it into pictures or through video format or through the information posted along with the picture

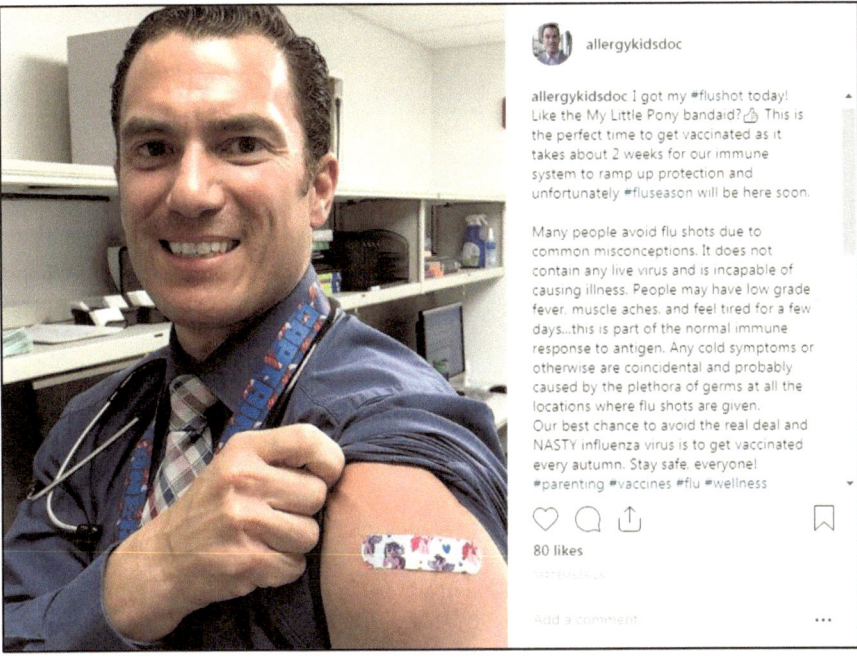

Fig. 1.7 Use of Instagram to disseminate health-related information. (Adapted from https://www.instagram.com/allergykidsdoc/)

(Fig. 1.7). Some downsides attributed to Instagram include the potential for cyberbullying through the comments feature, pictures and videos being posted that depict illicit drug use or nudity, and censorship with removal of accounts deemed inappropriate.

Instagram for Healthcare Professionals

Due to the nature of Instagram as a photo and video sharing platform with inability to provide easy access to links for websites or other information, it is not typically the primary social media platform used by healthcare professionals or organizations. However, the audience on Instagram can differ from Facebook and Twitter, so establishing an account and posting valuable content can reach different users and be used to drive traffic to other content or platforms. There are numerous examples of individual healthcare professionals who have established successful Instagram accounts by disseminating health-related information. This occurs by posting slides/photos/pictures discussing specific health-related information or by directly uploading videos that include the professional discussing a health-related topic. Other healthcare professionals use Instagram as a way to interact on a more personal level with followers while utilizing other social media platforms to disseminate health-related information. Professional organizations, practices, and hospitals can use

Instagram to build their online presence and post photos of patient success stories or efforts in the community.

Twitter

Twitter launched in 2006 and is the most used microblogging site, with over 500 million active users. Users establish profiles and accounts then can post short 280 character "Tweets" that can be shared with followers or the world at large. Posting a message is known as a tweet. Twitter allows users to connect with one another by following other people's Twitter feeds. When an account is followed, anything that account posts or retweets will appear in the timeline of the follower.

One of the most interactive parts of Twitter is the retweet feature. Retweeting allows users to repeat, or resend, tweets from other users. Tweets can be purely retweeted, which maintains their original message, including the account name and profile picture of the original tweeter, or comments can be added by the account doing the retweeting, which will still include the original tweet but now allows for sharing opinions or information directly related to the retweet. Retweeting is how information on Twitter is shared rapidly among large numbers of followers and users and is the central element to making tweets go "viral."

Twitter takes advantage of hashtags, which are common words or phrases preceded by a "#" symbol. This links all tweets using the same hashtag into the same search and also enters into the Twitter algorithm that decides which hashtags or topics are trending (garnering the most engagement) during a particular time frame or by location (see Chap. 6 for a more in depth discussion). Hashtags are very popular among professional organizations during their annual conferences. Use of a common hashtag (which is predetermined by the organization) from tweets originating from conference sessions allows attendees to link their tweets into the same timeline and also allows non-attendees to follow information being disseminated from within the conference. This raises the profile of the professional organization and can result in large spikes in tweeting activity during the conference, not to mention media inquiries. Peer-reviewed publications have originated from multiple specialties surrounding the concept of "Tweeting the meeting," including data demonstrating wide engagement, increased use of Twitter over the past few years, and review articles outlining best practices for organizations and attendees [10, 11].

Tweets are sent immediately and can spread across the world in a matter of seconds. This feature has led Twitter to be a major source of late breaking news. Many users turn to Twitter to learn the latest information pertaining to everything from natural disasters to traffic updates or celebrity breakups. Similar to short messages sent via text messaging, Twitter sends short messages to the entire platform. As discussed earlier, the rapid nature of information sharing that occurs through Twitter, along with the limitations in length of each post, can create rapid sharing of opinions and emotional responses, which may not reflect a measured and thoughtful reply. Twitter is a very public forum and while users can make their accounts private, by and large, users join Twitter to interact with a wide audience from across the world.

Unfortunately, many users forget that anyone can see their tweets, and once they hit send, it is out there forever. Even when original tweets are deleted, they may have been retweeted or captured by screen shot to live indefinitely. There are countless examples of professionals, athletes, celebrities, and politicians facing backlash from posts to their personal Twitter account years before they became famous. A recent example involves the actor/comedian Kevin Hart. On December 5, 2018, Kevin Hart was announced as the host for the 2019 Oscars presentation, scheduled to take place 2 months later. Within 24 hours, the Oscars faced mounting backlash from various groups over homophobic prior standup material and tweets that Kevin Hart posted in 2010. He had previously apologized for his words and actions, but everything surfaced again 8 years later, even after his previous tweets had been deleted. Within 48 hours of the original announcement, Kevin Hart stepped down as host of the Oscars due to the surging backlash [12]. This is one of countless examples demonstrating the same lesson: once you hit "send" on a tweet, it is out there forever.

The dark side of Twitter involves cyberbullying. Due to its instantaneous and viral nature, mean-spirited messages can be tweeted at users very easily and repeated over and over again. Twitter accounts can be anonymous or a false misrepresentation, so users may have no idea who is sending nasty messages their way. Twitter

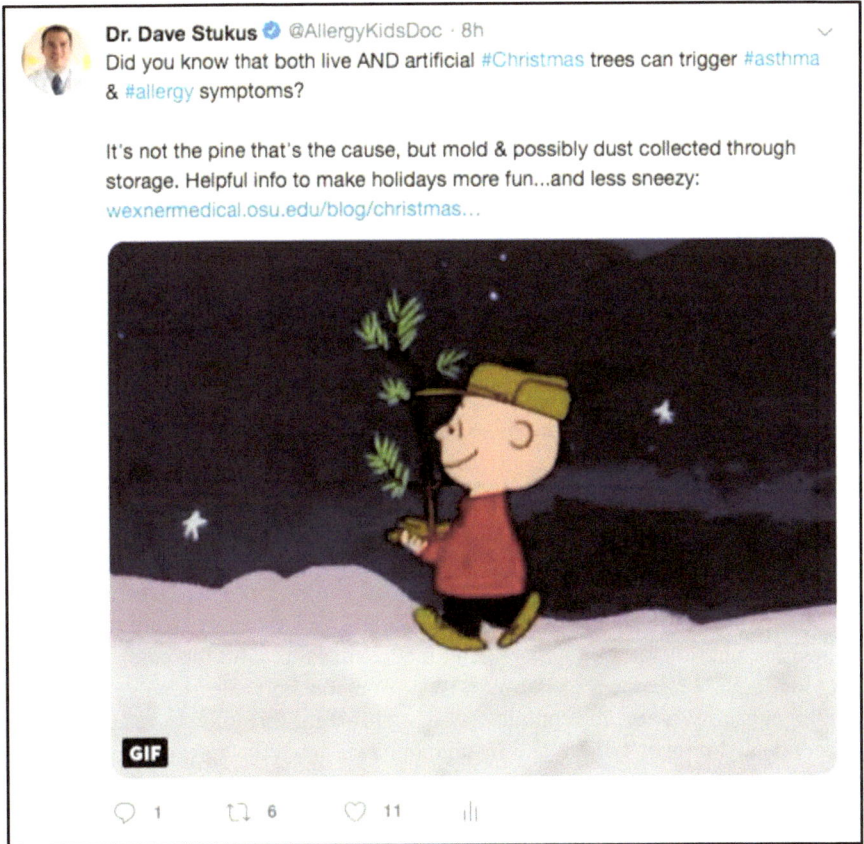

Fig. 1.8 Use of GIFs, hashtags, and links to websites for additional information can make tweets more noticeable and engaging. (Adapted from https://twitter.com/AllergyKidsDoc)

has incorporated a "block" feature that can prevent abusive accounts from seeing any information posted by the user. Accounts can also be "reported" to Twitter for review of their practices and consideration of suspension of their account. The notifications feature of Twitter allows users to see every reply, comment, retweet, and like of their posts. This can be dangerous territory if a user is sending tweets of a controversial or emotional nature, which naturally attract opinionated replies and comments. However, it also serves as a useful way to monitor those that retweet one's content and can lead to constructive interaction and network building.

Twitter is a popular way to share information very rapidly to a wide-reaching audience. Links to articles and online resources can be included within tweets, as long as the character limit is not exceeded (Fig. 1.8). Photos, GIFs, and videos can be linked to tweets, making them more entertaining and noticeable. Access to high-profile celebrities and politicians is an enticing aspect to Twitter for many users. Sitting Presidents of the United States have used Twitter to post their thoughts and opinions, which allows immediate unfiltered access to the leader of the free world.

Twitter for Healthcare Professionals

Twitter has widely become adopted as a prominent channel for healthcare professionals to disseminate health-related information, research findings, media stories, and information from meetings. Professionals interact with one another, answer questions, and network with colleagues from across the world. Most health-related professional organizations have Twitter accounts to serve as conduits for their members and the general public. Medical journals use Twitter to post online articles and hold virtual journal clubs. Twitter has been used successfully to promote advocacy efforts and mobilize physicians for a common cause. For instance, the American Academy of Pediatrics has a robust presence on Twitter and uses common hashtags to mobilize their pediatrician members surrounding issues related to healthcare reform, child welfare, and anti-vaccine sentiments. For healthcare professionals who are interested in getting more involved in social media and growing their online presence, Twitter offers a fast lane to making connections, growing an audience, and learning from like-minded colleagues.

Reddit, Snapchat, Pinterest...The List Goes On and On

There are multiple other popular social media sites that have the potential to reach a wide target audience. For the purposes of healthcare professionals or organizations engaging with the public or disseminating health-related information, Facebook, YouTube, Twitter, and Instagram have shown the most traction and value thus far. However, creative minds can always tap into new resources and avenues to achieve similar goals. The first question I'm sure many are asking is: Who has all the time? This subject will be addressed in greater depth in Chap. 3, but the point is valid. It is likely most productive to concentrate on one or two social media platforms, especially at first, and gain a following through dedicated efforts to those sites rather than cast a wide net and struggle with finding the time to maintain engagement on each site. At the very least, it is worthwhile for healthcare professionals to be aware of the variety of social media offerings, not only for their own use and professional purposes, but also for their patients, aquaintances and children, who will undoubtedly be using some of these platforms.

Reddit's site bills itself as the "front page of the Internet." With over 300 million users, it rivals Twitter in regard to reach. Reddit acts as a collection of forums, allowing users to share news, content, or comment on other posts. The "subreddits" within Reddit are smaller communities organized by topic, which assists navigation. The organization of the forum and language used by Reddit can be confusing at first. The home page displays posts that are trending on the site and are cultivated from a variety of subreddits. There are sort and search features to help users find content of interest. A unique feature of Reddit is the ability for users to upvote or downvote posts by clicking arrows on each post, which results in increasing or decreasing the visibility of each post. Each Reddit account has a "karma" number associated with it, which indicates how much karma their comments have accumulated. A user's karma score can boost standing within the Reddit community. Essentially, Reddit offers a forum for posting content and promotes interaction and discussion through various features. Healthcare professionals could utilize Reddit to create their own subreddit community and post health-related information or to post/comment on other user's posts.

Snapchat is a photo and video sharing service similar to Instagram and has gained popularity among younger generations. Snapchat has almost 200 million users and bills itself as a "new kind of camera that's connected to your friends and the world." The most unique feature of Snapchat is that photos and videos (called snaps) are meant to disappear after they're viewed. It acts as a camera by allowing users to take a picture or video; add filters, lenses, or other effects; and then share them with their network of friends. Videos can be up to 10 seconds in duration, and snaps can be added to a user's Story, which is very similar to Instagram and lasts 24 hours before disappearing. The nature of Snapchat makes it a difficult forum for disseminating information, providing links, or having discussions related to healthcare information. Instead, it is designed to be a fun way for people to connect and share moments from their lives with friends and family.

Pinterest is similar to Instagram and Snapchat with a focus on pictures and visual content. Pinterest acts like a web-based bulletin board and bookmarking tool. Users can "pin" or save images from other sites to different boards utilized to categorize information. The images can be clicked and then open to a new tab with links to the original web page. As such, Pinterest has become a very popular tool for sharing recipes, which allows users to scroll through images of meals and food and then click on links to the recipes used to create these colorful masterpieces. Pinterest incorporates elements of social networking as users can like other pins, leave comments, and re-save other user's content. Private messaging is another feature that encourages user interaction and networking. The ability to click pictures to open longer format links lends itself to potential use for healthcare professionals, especially if trying to reach a different audience than found on other social media platforms. Pinterest could be used to generate interest through pictures or infographics, direct users to additional health-related content, and then generate discussion through comments. It could also be used for advocacy or raising awareness to public health information.

LinkedIn and Doximity

LinkedIn and Doximity are the two most widely used professional social media sites. These are designed to be used by professionals as a way to provide an online presence for individuals and promote networking. LinkedIn is described as the "World's Largest Professional Network" and has over 300 million registered users. LinkedIn affords an opportunity for users to highlight their professional achievements, and many view it as an abridged curriculum vitae. The profile page on LinkedIn offers a quick glance at one's educational profile and can be as detailed as one likes. Many professionals view LinkedIn as a necessity for maintaining control over their individual content (unlike online physician rating sites, for instance), assisting Google search results, connecting with those who have similar interests, posting of articles, and assisting recruitment and employment opportunities. The benefit of LinkedIn, as opposed to Facebook, is the devotion to professional-only content and does not include personal information. Some downsides of LinkedIn include a fee for more premium services and a voyeuristic side that allows users to see who has looked at their profile, followed by site-derived suggestions for who to connect with based upon these clicks.

Doximity is very similar to LinkedIn and is often referred to as "LinkedIn for doctors," but unlike LinkedIn, it is only available for healthcare professionals located in the United States. This site focuses on physician engagement (with recent additions for nurse practitioners, physician assistants, and pharmacists) and allows for user profiles to highlight educational and professional accomplishments. Doximity also offers Continuing Medical Education, HIPAA-compliant email, text and faxing, and a news portal. A unique feature of Doximity is the ability to convert faxes into digital messages that can be sent to another user, which is useful when requesting records from other offices or hospitals. One downside of Doximity is that the site can create profiles for physicians, even if they have not claimed their own site. Doximity pre-populates information based upon databases, and it is up to each user to "claim" their profile, which then allows them to edit and upload new content. Users can upload their curriculum vitae, provide information regarding their practice and services offered, add press mentions, and enable a feature to automatically upload press mentions. Physician profiles are searchable and available to the public.

Conclusion

This introductory chapter introduced basic concepts surrounding social media and the various platforms that can be used by healthcare professionals. Social media has dramatically changed how information is disseminated and shared among individuals. For the first time in history, humans from across the world are connected with one another in real time, allowing them to share their personal information, thoughts, and ideas. As we all learn how to best navigate this evolving experience, we must remain aware of the potential benefits as well as risks. The remaining chapters will address specific aspects of social media pertaining to engagement and growing an audience, provide a blueprint for healthcare professionals with practical tips to either get started or continue to grow an online presence, and hopefully motivate many more to get more involved.

References

1. Markham MJ, Gentile D, Graham DL. Social media for networking, professional development, and patient engagement. Am Soc Clin Oncol Educ Book. 2017;37:782–7.
2. Greenwood S, Perrin A, Duggan M. Social media update 2016. Pew Research Center, 11 Nov 2016. www.pewinternet.org/2016/11/11/social-media-update-2016/.
3. Gottfried A, Shearer E. News use across social media platforms 2016. Pew Research Center, 26 May 2016. www.journalism.org/2016/05/26/news-use-across-social-media-platforms-2016/.
4. International smartphone mobility report. Informate Mobile Intelligence, Mar 2015. https://www.prnewswire.com/news-releases/no-time-to-talk-americans-sendingreceiving-five-times-as-many-texts-compared-tophone-calls-each-day-according-to-new-report-300056023.html.
5. Murdock KK. Texting while stressed: implications for students' burnout, sleep, and well-being. Psychol Pop Media Cult. 2013;2(4):207.
6. Bansal A, Garg C, Pakhare A, Gupta S. Selfies: a boon or bane? J Family Med Prim Care. 2018;7(4):828–31.
7. 2014–2016 Ebola outbreak in West Africa. https://www.cdc.gov/vhf/ebola/history/2014-2016-outbreak/index.html. Accessed 6 Dec 2018.
8. Most popular social networks worldwide as of July 2018, ranked by number of active users (in millions). Statista. Accessed 7 Dec 2018.
9. Youtube.com. Traffic, demographics and competitors. www.alexa.com. Accessed 7 Dec 2018.
10. Djuricich AM, Zee-Cheng JE. Live tweeting in medicine: 'tweeting the meeting'. Int Rev Psychiatry. 2015;27(2):133–9.
11. Pemmaraju N, Mesa RA, Majhail NS, Thompson MA. The use and impact of Twitter at medical conferences: best practices and Twitter etiquette. Semin Hematol. 2017;54(4):184–8.
12. How Kevin Hart tweeted himself out of a job hosting the Oscars. https://www.theverge.com/2018/12/8/18131221/kevin-hart-oscar-hosting-homophobia-twitter-tweets. Accessed 8 Dec 2018.

A Brief History of Digital Communications

2

Michael D. Patrick

> *During my service in the United States Congress, I took the initiative in creating the internet.*
>
> —Vice President Al Gore

In the Beginning...

Al Gore did not create the Internet – that had come much earlier, in 1968. However, he did play a critical role in shaping the Internet into the enormous, global collection of information we know today. Anyone with a computer or smartphone can freely explore any topic, including all things medical, on websites, social media, blogs, YouTube, podcasts, and mobile apps. But it hasn't always been this way. Our digital way of life did not fall into our laps haphazardly. A multitude of pioneers played important roles in creating these digital resources, and those seeking medical information took advantage of their work every step of the way.

To understand how we got here, let's travel back to 1968. Engineers at BBN Technologies, a private company in Cambridge, Massachusetts, were working on a new project funded by the US Department of Defense Advanced Research Project Agency (ARPA). BBN began as an acoustics consulting company in 1948, and their first contract was an important one: helping design the sound characteristics of the United Nations Assembly Hall in New York City. Their work required complex calculations, which led the company to invest in the newly expanding field of computer science by the late 1950s. BBN pioneered the use of computer models to design noise barriers around airports and highways and to design acoustically pleasing concert spaces, such as MIT's Kresge Auditorium and Lincoln Center's Avery Fisher Hall. By the mid-1960s, the company had acquired an impressive collection of computers, which was no small feat given the cost and size of each machine.

© Springer Nature Switzerland AG 2019
D. R. Stukus et al., *Social Media for Medical Professionals*,
https://doi.org/10.1007/978-3-030-14439-5_2

ARPA approached BBN because the Department of Defense also owned a collection of computers and was interested in connecting the machines together over great distances to send communications. This was an easy task with two machines connected by wire, but adding a third created problems – how could the computers form a network? How could one machine choose another, send a private message, and hide it from the other?

The answer came in 1968, when BBN developed the "Interface Message Processor" (IMP) in a metal box the size of a soda machine. This first network router would assign a digital address to three computers and direct messages between them. The team wanted computers connected from different sites and enlisted the help of three universities: UCLA, Stanford, and UC Santa Barbara.

At 10:30 pm on the night of October 29, 1969, Charlie Kline fired up a computer at UCLA and sent a message to Bill Duvall at Stanford. This first message transmitted over a digital network were the letters "LO." Charlie had aimed to send "LOGIN," but the first network crash also came the evening of October 29, cutting his message short. Moments later, the team rebooted the system, and Charlie and Bill began sending text messages back and forth across the network, one character at a time [1].

Over the next 2 years, the team employed additional IMP routers and connected 20 computers to the network. These machines were hosted by academic institutions and government agencies on the West Coast. In 1970, ARPANET crossed the continental United States when BBN connected their Massachusetts headquarters to the network. Schools on the Atlantic seaboard and upper Midwest soon followed; and in 1973, the network grew across the Atlantic with a satellite link to computers in Norway and an underwater cable connection to London. In 1975, the US Department of Defense declared ARPANET "operational" and took control of the project. However, additional academic institutions and government agencies continued to join, and the military limited their use of the network to unclassified communications.

Over the next decade, ARPANET deployed more IMP routers as hundreds of universities joined the network. Meanwhile, additional North American networks began springing up, along with networks in Europe and Australia. Gateways between ARPANET and these other systems would slowly give rise to the global Internet we know today.

In addition to expanding reach, ARPANET also grew in capability. In the beginning, communication was limited to strings of characters forming simple text messages. This gave rise to increasingly complex protocols that allowed the transmission of files. Protocols could convert the content of a document into a set of instructions that could be transmitted across the network and used by the receiving computer to recreate the content. Initially, files were limited to text documents, but as technology and protocols advanced, sending more complicated files across the network became possible. The advent of file transfer protocol (FTP) in 1971 led to the sharing of spreadsheets, images, and sounds. Unfortunately, individual networks developed different sets of protocols, making it difficult to communicate and send files from one network to another. A standard protocol was needed, and the Transmission Control Protocol/Internet Protocol (TCP/IP) eventually won the job. ARPANET adopted TCP/IP in 1983 and virtually all other networks quickly followed suit. TCP/IP continues driving data across the Internet today.

Compu-Serv

ARPANET immediately caught the eye of the private sector. One company with an interest in computer connectivity was the Golden United Life Insurance Company, headquartered in Columbus, Ohio. Many of their field offices housed a computer, and in an effort to create their own network, Golden United acquired a router in 1969. In addition to conducting business between offices, Golden United began offering a collection of interesting digital documents to share, including news articles, stock prices, and weather forecasts. Local residents began visiting the insurance company, not to buy a policy, but to use the computer to access this information. The company was happy to allow it but charged these customers by the minute. Using Golden United computers became so popular that the company purchased additional routers and began allowing home users and other businesses to connect to their network with a modem and telephone line. The model was profitable, and as their customer base grew, Golden United spun off a subsidiary known as the Compu-Serv Network, which would far outlive the company's insurance business [2].

Compu-Serv (later changed to CompuServe) dominated the commercial online service industry in the 1970s and 1980s by broadening their offerings and pioneering public access to large volumes of digital documents, file transfers, bulletin boards, and electronic mail. Subscribers could login to their account from home and check TV listings, sports scores, and current events from around the world. In 1980, CompuServe partnered with the Associated Press and several newspapers, including *The Columbus Dispatch*, *The New York Times*, *The Washington Post*, and *San Francisco Chronicle*. However, reading an entire newspaper remained impractical because the text of a 20-cent print edition could take several hours to download at a connection cost of $5 per hour [3, 4].

Additional fee-for-service networks emerged in the 1980s, including Prodigy (1984) and General Electric's GEnie Network (1985). However, these commercial networks (including CompuServe) were isolated from one another and did not provide access to ARPANET or other global networks.

Reading an entire newspaper remained impractical because the text of a 20-cent print edition could take several hours to download at a connection cost of $5 per hour.

Usenet and Newsgroups

Prior to the digital revolution, those searching for medical information outside the doctor's office had limited options. Libraries and book stores supplied self-help volumes, and magazine articles offered additional expert advice. Local support groups provided assistance; and, of course, friends and relatives offered sought-after as well as unsolicited counsel. However, finding the answer to a specific question could prove difficult, with reliability of answers dependent upon the small number of available resources.

Network connections opened the lines of communication between strangers, both laypersons and medical experts, in a way that had not been possible before.

This began in earnest with the creation of discussion forums and bulletin boards on ARPANET and the commercial networks. CompuServe, in particular, grew a large community of moderated discussion forums centered around specific topics. Subscribers could join discussions on any number of areas, including politics, sports, computer science, health, and wellness. These forums consisted of single messages left as a thread and perpetually available for reading and commenting. Moderators facilitated each discussion, ensuring participants followed group rules and etiquette. Health and wellness discussions were popular and often centered around a specific disease or condition, such as diabetes, heart disease, or cancer. The quality of discussions varied greatly, depending on the makeup of the group, but in many instances experienced laypersons and medical professionals joined the conversation, offering practical advice and expert answers to specific questions.

Similar groups sprang up on ARPANET and other networks. Unmoderated bulletin boards and newsgroups also grew in popularity. These were similar to discussion forums in that threads of messages were left for all to see and add comment. However, users could start their own threads, and comments remained uncensored. There was a wild-west, anything-goes feeling to these groups, which included adult-oriented and sometimes pornographic conversations, especially on public unpoliced networks, such as ARPANET. Still, one could skim thousands of topics and join what seemed to be a global conversation. Medical advice was no longer limited to office visits, books, magazines, friends, and neighbors. You could pose a question to the network and receive an answer (perhaps reliable, perhaps not) within a matter of minutes. The world of medical information sharing was truly changing!

Tom Truscott and Jim Ellis were graduate students at Duke University in 1979 when they conceived an unmoderated bulletin board/newsgroup system for students and faculty at Duke and the University of North Carolina at Chapel Hill. They established a hierarchal system of threads that could easily be indexed and searched. Science-related topics were categorized under the sci.* heading, with threads related to medicine, health, and wellness listed under sci.med.* and alt.health.*. They launched the system as Usenet in 1980; and because the universities connected with ARPANET, a large number of users accessed the system. Rather than hosting Usenet on a single computer, Tom and Jim established an army of "Usenet servers" that could communicate with each other over the network and update content as it was added. In this way, a user could add comments to one server and see those comments eventually replicated among all the other servers. Thus, Usenet became a reliable information repository immune to computer crashes or intentional shut down by a single institution or organization [5].

As the database grew, developers created software programs known as "newsreaders." These could access Usenet servers from a variety of computing platforms, allowing users to subscribe to specific threads, mark comments as "read," and provide notification when new remarks arrived. This made it easier to stay current on a specific topic, including those related to health and wellness. Users could search for new threads, keep track of preferred conversations, and avoid wasting time scrolling through old comments.

Network Growth

The late 1970s brought a decline in funding for ARPANET, and the Department of Defense no longer had an interest in adding new connections. However, interest in joining a computer network remained high at many universities; and in 1981, the National Science Foundation (another agency of the US government) provided funding for a new network of academic institutions called the Computer Science Network (CSNET). Inaugural members of CSNET included the University of Delaware, Princeton, and Purdue. Within a few years, CSNET included an international collection of 180 academic institutions. This provided a means of digital communication between member schools, but the problem of isolation remained as faculty and students at CSNET schools were unable to communicate with their peers at ARPANET schools.

In 1985, the National Science Foundation created a second network. They recruited five sites across the United States to host supercomputers and increased transmission speed among them from 2.4 kilobits per second (kbit/s) to 56 kbit/s. This collection of connected supercomputers, known as the National Science Foundation Network (NSFNET) included a gateway, hosted by BBN Technologies in Massachusetts. The NSF invited other networks to connect through this gateway as long as the network could send and receive data at the higher transmission rate. ARPANET, CSNET, and many commercial and private networks jumped at the opportunity by updating their transmission technology and tapping into the system. In this way, the NSFNET emerged as the first real widespread network of networks.

Meanwhile, the size and cost of personal computers began to shrink. This meant more institutions, businesses, and homes were connecting to a network and moving digital data through NSFNET. By 1987, network traffic was always congested, and the National Science Foundation searched for a solution that would move data in a more efficient manner. This led to the development of 11 nodes within the network that could achieve higher bandwidth. Each node consisted of a supercomputer that communicated with other nodes at speeds of 1.5 Megabits per second (Mbit/s). These high-speed connections represented a 25-fold increase in transmission capacity and became known as the "T-1 backbone."

The T-1 backbone was like an interstate highway system for digital data. Users would connect from home, office, or school through a slow congested network, only to be whisked off through high-speed lines before reaching the final destination by way of another slow connection. The end result, however, was improved speed, efficiency, and reliability.

Traffic across the T-1 backbone doubled every 7 months, and network engineers estimated overload would return by 1990. In an effort to prevent this, NSF enlisted the help of several private corporations, including IBM and MCI, to build a new T-3 backbone, which would carry data between 16 supercomputer nodes at speeds of 45 Mbit/s. This new backbone entered service in 1991, just as a new type of data transmission, hypertext transfer protocol (http), began to see use [6].

The Internet and World Wide Web

The term "Internet" was first coined in the 1970s as work began on data transmission protocols. Any network using the TCP/IP set of protocols was considered to be an "Internet" even though these networks were not physically connected. The name began to catch on around the time ARPANET connected to NSFNET and was used to describe the growing collection of networks connecting through the NSF gateway at BBN Technologies. In 1990, Ed Kroll, a network manager at the University of Illinois Urbana-Champaign, published a list of every IP address and domain name connected through NSFNET. He called his document the "Internet Manager's Phonebook." This cemented the notion that NSFNET and its collection of connected networks made up the "Internet." Ed would go on to author The Hitchhiker's Guide to the Internet, one of the first self-help manuals for understanding and using this growing network of networks.

Personal home computers grew in popularity during the late 1980s, following the release of Apple's Macintosh Operating System (Mac OS) in 1984 and Microsoft Windows in 1985. Home users could engage digital content easily with software programs and network connections. However, during this time, network content remained text-based or individual image files that users downloaded before viewing. In 1990, Tim Berners-Lee, an English Scientist with the European Organization for Nuclear Research in Switzerland, and Robert Cailliau, a computer scientist from Belgium, proposed a system of network computer "servers" containing "pages" of text that included "hyperlinks." These pages were written in a language called "hypertext markup language" (html) and transmitted from one computer to another by way of "hypertext transfer protocol" (http) overlying a TCP/IP connection. These pages of text could be viewed by a computer-based "browser," which would locate a page using a network address called a Uniform Resource Locator (URL). The browser could then read the page and display its content. The network address of the server would consist of the customary string of numbers. However, words could be typed into the browser, which would be converted to the numerical address by a "name server," running on the network. Certain words on the page represented hyperlinks; which, when activated, would launch the browser to another page on a different server. They called this hypertext project the "World Wide Web."

Within months of their proposal, researchers had an operational service, but web servers and pages were limited to computers housed within the Cluster of European Research Projects (CERP). The team welcomed research sites outside of CERP in January 1991 and with the Internet at large in August. The first web server outside of Europe began service in December 1991 at the Stanford Linear Accelerator Center in Palo Alto, California.

Over the next 2 years, html advanced to include stylized text and images, but available browsers could not read the updated language, and most web pages remained simple text. Internet traffic to web servers remained low, with users favoring Usenet and file transfer protocol applications such as Gopher. A breakthrough occurred in 1993 when Marc Andreessen and his team at the National Center for Supercomputing Applications (NCSA) at the University of Illinois at

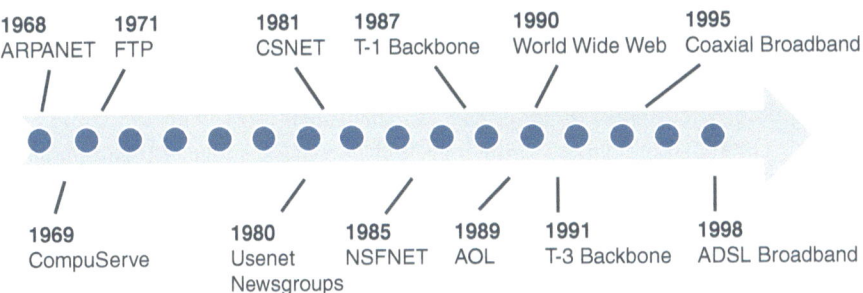

Fig. 2.1 Timeline of Internet milestones

Urbana-Champaign developed a graphical browser called "NCSA Mosaic." This browser could display stylized text and images, much like the content of a newspaper, magazine, or book. The team developed versions of their software compatible with Macintosh OS and Microsoft Windows, opening the World Wide Web to the rapidly growing base of home computer users [7].

Funding for the Mosaic Project was provided by the US High-Performance Computing and Communications Initiative and the High-Performance Computing Act of 1991, which were introduced to Congress by Senator Al Gore. This legislation sought to bring disjointed public and private networks together, upgrading their technology and connecting them to the NSFNET T-3 backbone. It provided funds for strengthening national networking infrastructure and developing new web technologies. Al Gore envisioned a digitally connected world, which shared a vast library of information with speed and ease. He brought the term "information superhighway" into the public's vocabulary; and, although Al Gore did not "invent" the Internet, he did play a critical role in advocating for network research and development and securing the funds needed to achieve our digital age. See Fig. 2.1 for a visual representation of major milestones.

Advanced Browsers and the Rise of Websites

After the Mosaic Project closed, Marc Andreessen and fellow computer scientist and entrepreneur, Jim Clark, started a company called Netscape, which developed and released Netscape Navigator in 1994 [8]. This browser was more polished with an array of advanced features, including displaying websites as they loaded rather than waiting for the entire page to download before displaying text and images. Since home users dialed into the Internet through slow connections over telephone lines, this solved the problem of staring at a blank screen while waiting for a page to completely load. Netscape offered their Navigator free for noncommercial use, and the software quickly became the most popular web browser on the Internet. Microsoft released their version of a web browser, Internet Explorer, the following year, and the companies began to battle for the heart of users by adding an array of competitive features, including tabbed windows to display multiple pages at once and cookies to remember user data from one site visit to the next. In 1998, Netscape spun off a new company called the Mozilla Foundation, which released a new open-source browser. Those savvy in computer programming could tinker with the software, develop customized "plug-ins" and share their work with the world. This browser morphed into Firefox, which continues to be a popular web browser today [9]. Rounding out the modern browsers are Apple's Safari, introduced in 2003 and Google Chrome in 2008.

The advancement of browsers coincided with an explosion of websites, and the late 1990s brought a host of options for those wishing to create a web presence. Services like GoDaddy (1997) allowed affordable domain name registration and the required server space for hosting a site. Those without knowledge of html could use a "what you see is what you get" (WYSIWYG) editor to translate a specific design into the html code needed to reliably display the page in a browser. By 1998, there were 2.4 million websites, a dramatic increase from 2738 websites when Navigator released 4 years earlier.

The rise in websites brought more information into homes than ever before. Websites catering to a variety of topics and interests sprang up, creating a global open-access encyclopedia. Of course, the quality and reliability of information provided was only as good as its source, and since anyone with a little creative ingenuity could design and launch a website, the potential for myths and misconceptions to spread became as great as the potential to share reliable and useful information.

Several medical organizations and practicing physicians were early adopters of digital technology, offering free health and wellness websites to Internet users. The American Cancer Society hosted one of the first and largest of these websites at cancer.org (1994) where the latest information and research was made available to patients, medical providers, and researchers.

In 1995, Dr Alan Greene, a pediatrician in San Mateo, California, launched DrGreene.com. According to the American Medical Association, this was "the pioneer" physician website. Dr Greene provided answers to common questions and published articles on a variety of pediatric-related topics. In doing so, he was able to reach far beyond the walls of his practice and impact the health and wellness of children around the world.

The Nemours Foundation also launched a website in 1995 at KidsHealth.org. This sought to be a broadly based online encyclopedia of pediatric medical knowledge with the later development of four sub-sites aimed at particular populations, including young patients, teenagers, parents, and educators. In this way, the organization could present health information in language that was understandable and useful to a specific audience of web users.

In 1997, the Mayo Clinic launched a medical website providing health and wellness information for adult patients; and in 1998, Internet entrepreneur, Jeff Arnold, launched WebMD, a commercial site that displayed paid advertising alongside medical articles and images. WebMD grew to include symptom checkers, medication look-ups, and a growing collection of self-help offerings written by physicians with specific areas of expertise.

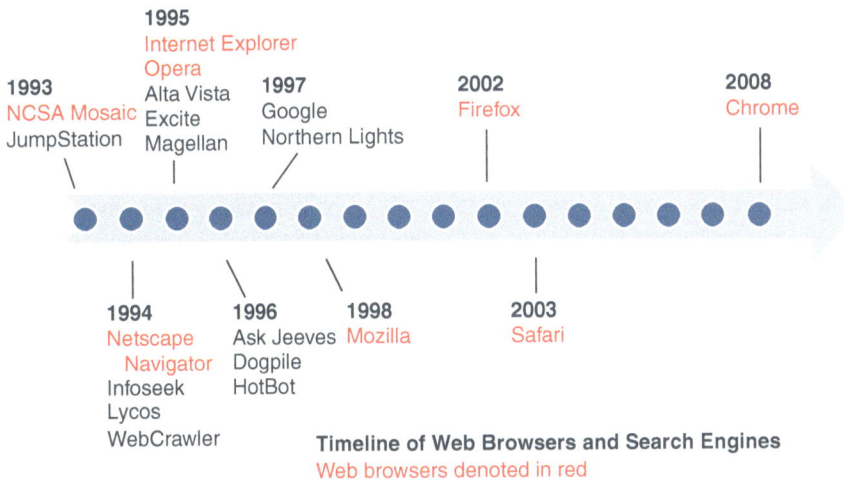

Fig. 2.2 Timeline of web browser development

Many new medical websites sprang up in the late 1990s, including drugs.com and Medline in 1998 and the Student Doctor Network, ePocrates, and Medscape in 1999. By the early 2000s, a growing library of digital medical content, spanning a vast range of specialties and catering to both the general public and medical professionals, was freely accessible from anywhere in the world. Al Gore's vision of an information superhighway was being realized, and those seeking medical information had many digital options for finding answers to their questions. See Fig. 2.2 for a timeline depiction of browser development.

America Online

As information permeated the Internet, the number of users accessing that information also grew. The decreasing cost and rising popularity of home computers placed a terminal capable of reaching the Internet in many homes and workplaces. Still, users would need to subscribe and connect with an online service to make Internet access possible. The successful Internet provider would need to be readily available, affordable, and easy for computer novices to use. America Online fit that bill for many computer owners.

The company began as Control Video Corporation in 1983, offering a service called GameLine. This allowed owners of the Atari 2600 gaming console to connect via telephone line and download games to the console for $1 per title. The game would remain until the user turned the console off or downloaded a new game. The company was not profitable and morphed into Quantum Computer Services in 1985. Quantum launched a networking product, similar to Compu-Serv, called Quantum Link, exclusively for users of Commodore computers [10]. It added new services to its portfolio, including AppleLink for Macintosh computers and PC Link for IBM PCs in 1988. The service differed from other online ventures at the time by offering software that provided more bells and whistles than a simple "dumb terminal" accessing online content. Users could chat across the network with a graphical interface, engage in interactive fiction, and play online games with other users running the same software.

In 1989, Quantum changed the name of its service to American Online (AOL). It introduced a version for Microsoft DOS in 1991 and Microsoft Windows in 1992. The service connected to Usenet in 1993 and began connecting with other Internet sites, such as National Geographic, the Smithsonian Institution, Library of Congress, and the National Education Association. AOL's software was the first to offer homework help, parental controls, and access to online courses. In 1996, AOL dropped its hourly connection rate and became the first commercial service to offer unlimited network access for a flat rate of $19.95 per month. AOL also launched an aggressive marketing campaign by including free AOL software CDs in mailers, magazines, and cereal boxes. At one point, 50% of all new CDs produced worldwide had an America Online logo [11]. This, combined with an introductory free month (or "100 hours of service"), led to millions of new subscribers. By mid-1997, half of all American homes with Internet access connected through AOL [12]. The following year, AOL purchased Netscape and began allowing subscribers unfiltered access to the World Wide Web through the Netscape browser.

The success of AOL led to significant connection problems. The company had trouble keeping up with the pace of new subscribers, and since users accessed the system using dial-up modems and land-based telephone lines, busy signals and long waits to connect were common. The other problem was speed. Dial-up modems could achieve a maximum speed of 56 kbit/s, meaning home users could not take full advantage of the blazing T-3 backbone. The popularity of surfing the web for information was gaining ground, but it remained a frustrating experience for many users. The world was ready for improved technology, connecting homes with the information superhighway via faster and more reliable onramps.

At one point, 50% of all new CDs produced worldwide had an America Online logo. By mid-1997, half of all American homes with internet access connected through AOL.

Physicians Online

As AOL gained traction, a similar service appeared, which catered to physicians. Launched in 1994, Physicians Online (POL) required doctors to verify their medical license before subscribing. Like America Online, POL used a dial-up connection and proprietary software. The company enticed subscribers to join by distributing floppy disks and CDs in journal mailings and at medical conferences. Clinicians could email one another and engage in medical (and nonmedical) conversations without the watchful eyes of patients and families. WebMD paid $2 million in cash for Physicians Online in 2003, citing the acquisition as a unique opportunity to connect a large community of verified doctors with the WebMD Medscape Health Network [13]. WebMD soon dropped the POL name and discontinued its desktop software and dial-up service in favor of their web-based product.

Broadband Connections

In 1996, the US Congress passed another important piece of legislation, the National Information Infrastructure Protection Act. This prioritized initiatives to build fast, reliable Internet connections for home users. Since most American homes were already wired with telephone lines and cable TV, these became the primary focus for improving Internet access.

Ordinary telephone lines are twisted pairs of copper wire, originally designed to deliver low-frequency analog voice signals between telephone handsets. Dial-up modems use these same low (and slow) frequencies to deliver data. Faster data transmission would require the use of high-frequency digital signals. Could ordinary telephone wires reliably transport these faster signals? This question was answered in the 1980s with the development of the Integrated Digital Services Network (ISDN). Businesses and communication companies began using ISDN in the late 1980s to deliver digital data, voice, and video signals over the traditional telephone network at speeds of 128 kbit/s. This allowed videoconferencing and the ability to send television signals between studios and transmission towers. In addition, ordinary telephone wire could carry these higher frequencies at the same time as low-frequency analog voice transmission, meaning the line could carry voice conversation and digital data at the same time.

The limiting factor for ISDN connections over ordinary telephone wire is distance. At about 2 miles, the signal decays and is no longer reliable. However, ordinary telephone wire is not used to connect neighborhoods with the phone company. Larger gauge wire, which transmits digital data faster and over longer distances, enters a neighborhood hub before splitting off to individual homes. As long as a home was within 2 miles from the hub, an ISDN connection could be made. Most homes were much closer than two miles to the closest hub, allowing an increase in speed. Additionally, ISDN technology advanced, allowing faster transmission with an asymmetric flow of data. This increased the downstream speed (from hub to home) at the expense of slower upstream speeds. This workaround was ideal for Internet users because the web tends to send more data than it receives.

In 1998, ISDN protocols were further modified, creating the asymmetric digital subscription line (ADSL), and telephone companies seized the opportunity to provide this high-speed service to homes. The first ADSL connections had a downstream rate of 384 kbit/s, which was seven times faster than a dial-up modem. ADSL has further improved over the years, with the introduction of ADSL2+ in 2008. This protocol can achieve speeds of 24 Mbit/s (430 times faster than dial-up) on the downstream path and 3.3 Mbit/s upstream.

The other wire entering most urban homes in the late 1990s transmitted cable TV. These "coaxial" cables contained a central core of thick copper surrounded by effective insulation. Because of this design, they are ideally suited to carry digital signals over long distances. Cable TV providers were eager to compete with telephone companies in developing technology to bring high-speed broadband connections to the American home. Time Warner Cable launched one of the first coaxial-based Internet connections in 1995 in Elmira, New York. They called this service the

Southern Tier On-Line Community [14]. It met great success, and the cable company began providing Internet access to additional neighborhoods with a service called LineRunner. As the product deployed to more cities, Time Warner adopted the cartoon character, Road Runner, as a mascot and changed the service name to Road Runner High Speed Online. Other cable companies were quick to follow suit, and the early 2000s saw an explosion of broadband options for American homes.

The speed at which coaxial cable transmits digital data is dependent on the type of line coming into a neighborhood hub, the number of residential users sharing the hub and the modem protocols employed. In the early days of cable Internet, 1 Mbit/s connections were common, providing 2–3 times faster speeds than ADSL from the same era. With the advent of fiber-optic cables to neighborhood hubs and improved modem technology, today's coaxial cable connections can generate downstream speeds greater than 1 gigabit per second (Gbit/s), which is 18,000 times faster than dial-up.

In 2000, broadband services were widely available in large urban areas, but the monthly rate was cost-prohibitive for many families. That year, only 3% of American homes subscribed to a broadband service, while 34% connected to the Internet with dial-up (63% had no Internet connection at all). However, by 2013, with decreasing cost and small-town availability, 70% of homes subscribed to broadband, and only 3% remained on dial-up [15].

High-speed Internet made it possible to bring increasingly complex websites to home users. Previously, those seeking medical information could discuss symptoms and diseases on bulletin boards, read the latest biomedical research in a newsgroup, or view X-rays and rashes on a website. High-speed Internet allowed much more. Users could interact with animated 3D renderings of the skeleton and organ systems, watch high-definition videos of the immune system in action, and visit the operating room to view the complicated steps of a surgical procedure. Internet connections were finally fast and efficient, without busy signals or network congestion (Table 2.1).

Table 2.1 History of Internet development and achievements

History of home network access		
Year	Service	Notable achievements
1969	CompuServe	First fee-for-service network access. Spin-off from the Golden Life Insurance Company in Columbus, Ohio
1984	Prodigy	First graphical user interface, making network access easy for novices
1985	Genie Network	Introduced multi-player online games. Refined bulletin boards and chat rooms
1989	America Online	Introduced unlimited service for a monthly fee. Provided 50% of home internet connections in 1997
1995	Road Runner	First coaxial broadband service. Introduced by Time Warner Cable as Southern Tier On-line Community
1998	ADSL Service	Broadband delivered by ordinary telephone wires Introduced by several regional phone companies
2007	Mobile Browsing	Apple's iPhone introduced the first fully functional mobile web browser for cellular and Wi-Fi connections

Search Engines

Prior to 1993, there were no automated search engines for the World Wide Web. Users could view manually created lists of available sites, but as waves of new offerings popped up, curators had difficulty keeping the lists current. Another problem related to content. Manually curated lists did not always reflect the nature or scope of information on a particular page, making searches for answers to specific questions difficult.

In 1993, Jonathon Fletcher, a computer scientist in England, created the first "web robot," called JumpStation [16]. This involved a computer server with code that automatically "crawled the web," looking for new sites. As sites were found, each was "indexed," meaning the program saved the website's address, title, and headings in a comprehensive database. Internet users could fill out a web form, which searched the database for specific words and returned a list of sites containing the query in a title or page heading. This setup provided an automatic system for keeping an updated list of websites and searching those sites based on titles and headings. However, JumpStation did not fully index the entire content of each site.

Brian Pinkerton launched a web robot at the University of Washington called WebCrawler in early 1994 [17]. This server indexed every word of a website, creating a more robust database that better reflected the content of the World Wide Web. WebCrawler became a popular Internet search tool and was purchased by America Online in 1995.

Each year brought new search engines with improved interfaces and additional features, including the ability to index graphics, videos, and Internet databases. Web robots became smarter, with the ability to detect changes in websites and update the database with fresh information. Search engines began ranking sites according to popularity and displayed profit-generating advertisements with their results. Popular entries included Infoseek and Lycos (1994); Magellan, Excite, and AltaVista (1995); Dogpile, HotBot, and Ask Jeeves (1996); and Northern Light (1997).

Although it wasn't a search engine, "Jerry and David's Guide to the World Wide Web" was another popular site for launching a search of the web. Jerry Yang and David Filo, electrical engineering students at Stanford University, launched this "human-edited" website directory in 1994 and changed the name to Yahoo the following year [18]. The pair wanted an easy-to-remember name; and David, who had grown up in Louisiana, suggested "Yahoo." The term had been widely used in his youth to describe an unsophisticated, rural southerner. They later devised a backronym for Yahoo: "Yet Another Hierarchically Organized Oracle," which described the organization of their site into many categories and subcategories [19]. By 1998, Yahoo was the most popular starting line for web surfers, beating out a plethora of available search engines. Yahoo did not attempt to include every website, only the best, at least in the opinion of site editors. Internet users appreciated their work, and many searchers of online medical information began their task of finding answers with Yahoo.

As Yahoo rose to prominence, another pair of Stanford students, Larry Page and Sergey Brin, embarked on another Internet project. They believed a search engine could return more relevant results if, in addition to indexing webpage content, the service also considered the number of "backlinks," meaning the sites that contained links to a particular page. The more backlinks to a page, and the more backlinks to each backlink, the more popular (and hopefully more useful) the page. They called this algorithm "PageRank," a nod to Larry's last name and the webpages they were ranking, and incorporated it into their Ph.D. Project, now called "BackRub."

BackRub would need more processing power than a typical search engine as it analyzed over 10 million webpages and the untold number of links between them. This bogged down Stanford's computer system, forcing the team to add additional servers made from spare computer parts, housed in cases made of Legos, and stacked inside a dorm room [20]. The search engine was first offered to the Stanford academic community, and the two students published a paper on their experience, "The Anatomy of a Large-Scale Hypertextual Web Search Engine," in the journal *Computer Networks* and ISDN Systems [21].

In 1997, Larry and Sergey opened their search engine to the entire World Wide Web and renamed it "Google," a reference to "googol," which is the number 1 followed by 100 zeros [22]. Google was an immediate hit, and by 1998 traffic was so great that Stanford kicked the project off their network. Larry and Sergey relocated the endeavor to an off-campus garage and obtained $100,000 in seed money from Andy Bechtolsheim, founder of Sun Microsystems [23]. Google's popularity continued to rise, and in 2000, Yahoo incorporated the search engine into their site, allowing users to explore the Yahoo directory or perform a Google search from the same starting place. Google also pioneered AdWords in 2000. This raised tremendous revenue as Google allowed businesses the opportunity to display advertisements alongside the search results of specific queries. Google has since grown into the most valuable provider of Internet-related products and services, with an estimated net worth of $279 billion US dollars in 2018 [24].

The pair wanted an easy-to-remember name; and David, who had grown up in Louisiana, suggested "Yahoo." The term had been widely used in his youth to describe an unsophisticated, rural southerner.

Advanced Web Programming Languages

If web browsers could read html code and translate strings of characters into stylized pages of words, images, and sounds, it stood to reason websites and browsers could learn to do even more. With creative ingenuity and cooperation between website developers and software engineers, programming languages emerged that allowed pages to come alive with engaging, interactive content. 1995 saw the first release of PHP, Ruby, and JavaScript. Macromedia Flash launched the following year. Advancement of these languages brought many new features to the web. Businesses offered online shopping carts and secure checkouts. Libraries served up digital versions of the card catalog and reserved books online, and medical websites created symptom checkers and drug-interaction tools.

Web programming languages gave Internet users the ability to securely change the content of a webpage on the fly. This eventually led to the development of blogs and social media sites. Until now, creating content for the World Wide Web had been a somewhat complex endeavor, requiring domain name registration, web-host server fees, expensive WYSIWYG software, or knowledge of html code. Programming languages allowed anyone with access to a computer and the Internet an opportunity to add their voice in an easy and accessible way. The information superhighway was about to explode with millions of content creators, each poised to engage in a global conversation. Our world would never be the same.

Blogs

Forums, newsgroups, and Usenet provided an opportunity for early Internet users to engage, debate, and share new ideas. The advent of blogging opened similar doors for millions of users on the World Wide Web; and with search engines indexing every blog page, users could find, read, comment, and engage on any topic and with any number of people around the world.

Jorn Barger, an avid Internet user from the United States, was a regular contributor of Usenet, with nearly 10,000 posts to his name by the mid-1990s [25]. As the web grew, Jorn explored thousands of sites and logged his discoveries on a self-created page called Robot Wisdom (1995) [26]. In 1997, he referred to this digital diary as a "web log." This morphed into "weblog," which soon became "blog." Others joined his rank with writings of their own, each finding a loyal audience of readers who were interested in some unique niche. These early bloggers blazed a new trail in digital publishing, one that required skills in website creation, but paid off with large audiences that rivaled articles published by traditional means.

In 1998, Bruce and Susan Ableson employed an advanced programing language and launched a website called Open Diary. This allowed Internet users the opportunity to create a blog without the usual steps of designing and hosting a website. Open Diary blogs were secure, and authors could edit content easily through their web browser. Readers left comments and engaged as a community, much like the early days of Internet bulletin boards. Additional blogging sites appeared, including Live Journal and Blogger in 1999. WordPress arrived in 2003 and has grown into the leading blog platform, hosting over 60 million sites by 2012 [27].

Blogs rose to prominence in the early 2000s. Early examples focused heavily on technology and political topics, but other interests were also represented. Dr. Jacob Reider, a family physician in New York, began one of the first medical blogs, DocNotes, in 1999 [28]. His primary audience was family physicians who enjoyed reading his commentary on medical technologies, small-town practice, wellness guidelines, and immunizations. Other health-related blogs followed, authored by medical professionals and laymen alike. Today, blogs can be found that support nearly any idea or point of view. Some are rooted in evidence, while others support less credible, yet persuasive, agendas.

RSS Feeds

One advantage newsgroups had over blogs was a convenient way of keeping track of interesting content. Newsreaders could flag threads of conversation and alert users to new messages, but keeping up with a collection of blogs proved more challenging. In 1999, Ramanathan Guha and Dan Libby, software engineers at Netscape, created the Rich Site Summary (RSS) [29]. RSS consists of a single text file, hosted on a web server. It keeps an updated account of the site's content, so when a new blog post is added, the RSS document is updated (either manually or through an automated process). Netscape introduced RSS functionality into their web browser, which allowed users to "subscribe" to "RSS feeds." Browsers could periodically check RSS files for new content and alert users when new posts became available. This allowed the web browser to function as a primitive newsreader.

Other web browsers incorporated RSS functionality and more sophisticated "RSS Readers" (apart from the web browser) became available. Now Internet users could subscribe to their favorite blogs and read the latest round of posts and comments with their morning cup of coffee. Blog authors encouraged readers to subscribe and engage in a way reminiscent of newsgroups, but on a grander scale. As more users subscribed to RSS feeds, a new acronym caught on: Really Simple Syndication.

Podcasts

As websites and blogs became the digital equivalent of books, newspapers, and magazines, it stood to reason downloaded audio files could stand in for music CDs and radio programs. Barriers to this development included the large size of audio files and slow connection speeds between home and the Internet, but as users embraced smaller, compressed mp3 audio files and broadband connections grew, the idea of sharing audio across the Internet became feasible. In 1999, Shawn Fanning and Shawn Parker launched Napster as a peer-to-peer file sharing service [30]. This used a web interface to copy a file directly from one home computer to another, without storing the file on a network server. This led to an explosion of (mostly illegal) music sharing and the growth of mp3 audio players. By 2001, with the arrival of Apple's iPod, many music lovers were trading in their cassettes, CDs, and Sony Walkman for this new digital technology.

2001 brought another development: the RSS "enclosure." This was an element of the RSS feed that notified subscribers when a new media file was added to a website. Bloggers could upload spoken audio or music files, and their followers could download the file and listen. This new form of communication was called "audioblogging." However, actual instances of audioblogging were rare, and most Internet users ignored the RSS enclosure.

This changed in 2004 when former MTV video jockey, Adam Curry, began recording a daily scripted radio-like program called *The Daily Source Code* [31]. Adam shared his personal life, commented on current events, played royalty-free music from a new website called the *Podsafe Music Network* and interviewed folks who had begun producing similar audio programs. Adam updated his RSS feed by adding a new enclosure with each episode release. Additionally, Adam encouraged his listeners to use an Apple computer script, known as iPodder, to automatically read his RSS feed, download new audio files to the computer and move the files into iTunes [31]. This process resulted in the delivery of new *Daily Source Code* episodes each time a listener plugged their iPod into the computer. These audio programs took on the name "podcasts" because they had been "broadcast" to an "iPod." In 2005, Apple incorporated RSS support in iTunes and published a directory of available shows. This new form of digital communication was now poised for significant growth.

The next 2 years saw the launch of many podcast programs, including medical ones. Listeners could get the latest health and wellness news, hear interviews with medical experts, and get their questions answered during the program. Early medical podcasts included content from The New England Journal of Medicine and Johns Hopkins University. PediaCast, from Nationwide Children's Hospital, introduced parents and pediatricians to podcasting, while New York University's Department of Ophthalmology pioneered continuing medical education credit by way of podcast.

Today's Internet user can access thousands of medical podcasts as they search for information online. From baby care to end-of-life issues and from family practice to narrowly focused subspecialties, listeners can learn from experts on nearly any health topic. Some shows target patients and families, while others cater to clinicians and researchers. Rather than replacing the traditional radio program, the audio podcast has far exceeded it, offering an encyclopedia of content-rich shows that were not possible before our digital revolution.

Social Networking Sites

Personal engagement among distant users has always been an integral part of the Internet, beginning with the first messages sent between UCLA and Stanford on ARPANET. Bulletin boards, newsgroups, blog posts, and podcasts encourage discussion on every imaginable topic, including those related to health and wellness. However, it was the arrival of social networking sites that fundamentally changed the way Internet users connect and communicate with one another.

These sites rely on advanced programming languages, massive databases, and modern browsers to grow enormous digital communities on the World Wide Web; and with over 2 billion active users [32], social media has single-handedly transformed the Internet into the widest-reaching communication platform in the history of man. Social media allows any individual the means to easily share information, thoughts, and ideas with those living down the street, across the country, and around the world.

Today's social networking sites can trace their beginning to a couple of online websites in the mid-1990s. Classmates Online (later known as Classmates.com) launched in 1995. Users could add specific schools, graduation years, work-places, and military units. As new people joined, they could find past affilia-tions and read brief profiles of long-lost friends. The site resembled a giant collection of yearbooks, but users could only send and receive messages if they purchased a "gold membership." Two years later, another website, SixDegrees.com, launched a more flexible service, rooted in the "six degrees of separation" concept, which states any two random people are connected through a series of six acquaintances. Users created an account and made a list of family, friends, and coworkers, regardless of any affiliations. Once added to a list, these acquaintances had the opportunity to confirm the relationship, join the website, and create a list of their own. Private messages could be freely sent among users, and bulletin board posts were visible to first-degree (friends), second-degree (friends of friends), and third-degree (friends of friends of friends) con-tacts. In this way, users could make new friends based on mutual connections. SixDegrees grew rapidly, attracting over three million subscribers between 1997 and 2000 [33].

Building on this idea, Jonathan Abrams, a computer programmer from Canada, launched another social networking site in 2002. He called the service Friendster, a combination of the words "friend" and "Napster," which was enjoying widespread popularity at the time [34]. Friendster introduced the "circle of friends" format of social networking. This entailed small virtual communities forming within the larger community, each based on a common user experience or interest. One might join communities associated with their former high school, favorite TV show, a popular video game, social stressor, or medical disease. Users looked up old friends and made new ones. Friendster surpassed SixDegrees in popularity, achieving over 100 million subscribers by 2008 [35].

Two important social media sites launched in 2003: MySpace and LinkedIn. MySpace catered to teenagers and young adults with an interest in pop culture and pioneered the individual "page" where users could share blog posts, photos, art, music, and videos. The service allowed users to connect with one another, form groups, send private messages, and adjust content filters and privacy settings. Like Friendster, MySpace achieved well over 100 million subscribers [36]; however, active users significantly declined by 2008 as Facebook became the dominant social media site [37]. LinkedIn launched as a professional networking site, connecting employers with job seekers. The service includes traditional social media functions, including connections with other users and the ability to share links, write blog posts, and send private messages. LinkedIn reported over 500 million registered users in 2017 [38].

The granddaddy of social networking sites, Facebook, can trace its beginnings to Harvard University and the dorm room of Mark Zuckerberg and Eduardo Saverin. Initially called FaceMash, the site launched in 2003 as a "hot or not" game for Harvard students [39]. The website stored a collection of female student pictures. Users of the site, which was limited to those on Harvard's network, were presented with two random pictures, side by side, and given the opportunity to decide who was hot and who was not. In its first 4 hours online, FaceMash served up 22,000 photos to 450 unique visitors [40].

Harvard administration frowned upon FaceMash and shut the site down after a few days of operation. Zuckerberg, who had written the code, faced expulsion. However, the university dropped charges, and Zuckerberg tweaked the code, replacing student photos with classic art and commentary. Fellow students could log on, add to the notes, and use the site as a study tool for the final examination of a popular art history class. When he returned to campus for Spring Semester, Zuckerberg modified the code further and created a Harvard student directory called "The Facebook." [41] Users could create a profile page with a picture of their choosing and message other users by writing on their "wall." The Facebook was announced through a campus mailing list, and within 24 hours of its launch, 1200 students joined [42].

In the Spring of 2004, The Facebook expanded, allowing students from Stanford, Columbia, and Yale. Ivy League and Boston area schools were added by summer, when Zuckerberg took The Facebook off the Harvard network and moved operations to Palo Alto, California. In 2005, "The" was dropped from the name and Facebook became available to every university in the United States, along with many large high schools and 21 colleges in the United Kingdom. By December 2005, Facebook reported nearly 6 million users [43]. The service had grown to include over 2000 colleges and 25,000 high schools throughout the United States, Canada, Mexico, the United Kingdom, Ireland, Australia, and New Zealand. Then, on September 26, 2006, Facebook opened its doors to anyone in the world 13 years of age or older with a valid email address. Within 2 years, in 2008, Facebook joined the ranks of Friendster and MySpace in attracting over 100 million users. However, the service would far outgrow these early social networking sites, climbing to 500 million users in 2010, 1 billion users in 2012 [43] and over 2 billion users in 2018 [32].

Facebook joined the ranks of Friendster and MySpace in attracting over 100 million users. However, the service would far outgrow these early social networking sites, climbing to 500 million users in 2010, 1 billion users in 2012 and over 2 billion users in 2018.

Meanwhile, another social networking platform, Twitter, also launched to the general public in 2006. This was the brainchild of Jack Dorsey, an undergraduate student at New York University and board member of a newly minted podcast company called Odeo. The board members were located in different parts of the country and desired a method of quick communication. Dorsey hired a contractor, Florian Weber, and the pair developed website code [44] and settled on the name Twitter because definitions of the word included "a short burst of inconsequential information" and "chirps from birds." With a limit of 140 characters per message, Twitter seemed an apt description of the service [45].

Twitter was initially limited to Odeo employees but opened to outside users within a few months. The service was quite different from other social networking sites in that all messages, called Tweets, could be read by any other user. However, one could fine-tune which messages showed up in their online "feed" by "following" a select group of other members. Within a year, Twitter users were sending over 20,000 tweets each day [46]. Awareness of the social platform grew during the 2007 South by Southwest Conference in Austin, Texas, thanks to the Twitter team

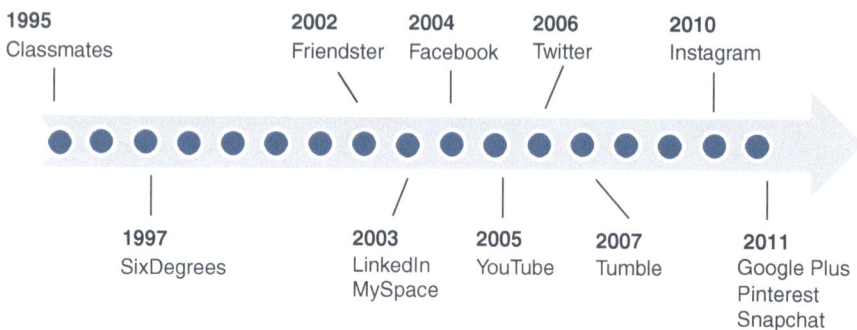

Fig. 2.3 Timeline of social media site development

moving two 60-inch plasma screens, each displaying moving feeds of tweets, around the meeting venue. The number of daily tweets spiked to 60,000 during the conference [46]. By 2010, Twitter users were sending 50 million tweets each day (about 750 tweets each second) [47]. This number increased to 200 million daily tweets in 2011 [48] and 500 million in 2013 [49]. While daily tweets plateaued at the 500 million mark between 2013 and 2018 [50], the number of monthly active users has grown from 204 to 335 million [51].

Additional social networking sites have made appearances, including YouTube (2005), Tumblr (2007), Instagram (2010), Google+ (2011), Pinterest (2011), and Snapchat (2011) (Fig. 2.3). All social networking sites provide tremendous opportunity for gathering medical information. Users can connect and support one another. Medical professionals and the general public coexist, asking questions, providing answers, and sharing resources, including links to websites, blog posts, podcasts, and videos.

Smartphones and Mobile Apps

The most recent development to impact the way we connect, communicate, and gather information is the rise of mobile technology. Smartphones can trace their beginning to the release of the first personal digital assistant (PDA) in 1984. The Organizer, introduced by the British company Psion, resembled a digital calculator with an expanded number of keys to include each letter of the alphabet. In addition to calculations, users could compose a digital diary and maintain a searchable database of telephone numbers and street addresses [52].

In 1986, Apple began developing a PDA platform known as the Newton [53]. First released in 1993, the device introduced the use of a touchscreen and stylus rather than a traditional alphanumeric keyboard. The Newton also pioneered handwriting recognition software, which allowed users to input letters and numbers with stylus strokes rather than pushing or tapping buttons. Unfortunately, the Newton did not gain consumer popularity, and Apple discontinued production in 1998 [54].

Palm Computing introduced their Palm Pilot PDA in 1996 [55]. The device built upon Apple's concept of using stylus strokes to input letters and numbers; however, compared to the Newton, the Palm Pilot was more affordable and easier to use. Sales were high and subsequent generations of Palm devices introduced new features, including backlit screens, color screens, expandable memory, and third-party software programs for the Palm Operating System. The latter gave Palm devices a genuine computer feel as users could accomplish tasks beyond taking notes and saving addresses. In 1999, the company introduced the Palm VII as the first PDA with a wireless connection to a limited number of Internet services and web pages.

As the PDA grew in popularity, cellular telephones became more affordable and smaller in size. By the late 1990s, many Americans had a PDA in one pocket and a cell phone in the other. Digital pagers were also popular (and often a requirement) of professionals, including those in the medical field. The time was ripe for a single device that could serve as telephone, PDA, and pager. RIM, a Canadian company, had this vision when they introduced the first Blackberry device in 1999 [56]. By 2002, the Blackberry could make phone calls, receive texts, check email, and browse simple websites. The smartphone, as we know it, had been born.

Despite the Blackberry's convergence of digital mobile technologies, the user experience was clumsy with input accomplished on an expansive array of physical buttons; and unlike Palm's devices, handwritten input and a robust collection of third-party software was missing. Two companies, Apple and Android, raced to develop a smartphone platform with Blackberry's feature set and Palm's ease of use and flexibility.

The result of Apple's work was the original iPhone, introduced in 2007 [57]. The company had expertise in both hardware and software development, and a loyal customer base poised to purchase 6.1 million iPhones in the first five quarters of production. Android was a software company and would need partnership with a manufacturing company to produce a physical smartphone. In the midst of their race with Apple, Google purchased Android and forged relationships with several manufacturing companies, including HTC, Motorola, and Samsung. The first Android-based smartphone, the HTC Dream (also known as the T-Mobile G1), debuted 1 year after iPhone in 2008 (Table 2.2) [58].

Table 2.2 History of smartphone development

History of personal digital assistants and smartphones		
Year	Product	Notable achievements
1984	The Organizer	First PDA. Users could maintain a diary and store telephone numbers and addresses
1993	Apple Newton	First PDA with touchscreen and stylus. Handwriting recognition converted screen strokes to text
1996	Palm Pilot	Improved stylus function and lower price. Subsequent models introduced third-party apps
1999	Palm VII	First PDA with wireless connection. Provided access to some internet services and web pages
1999	Blackberry	Combined features of PDA, telephone and pager. Relied on buttons rather than touchscreen
2007	Apple iPhone	First smartphone with stylus-free touchscreen, mobile web browser and large collection of third-party apps.
2008	HTC Dream T-Mobile G1	Introduced the Android operating system for smartphones

Ten years later, in 2018, over 2.5 billion people worldwide use smartphone devices [59]. Today's smartphone is a powerful pocket-sized computer with instant access to the Internet and a library of over 3 million available apps (software programs able to run on a smartphone's operating system) [60]. Smartphone users leverage their devices every day to connect, communicate, and share information in ways the first users of ARPANET could only dream of doing.

Conclusion

Our journey through the history of digital communication technology has come to an end. The cumulative result of this complicated sequence of events serves to benefits today's medical information seeker in an untold number of ways. Internet users can find the same evidence-based information available to medical students and practicing clinicians related to disease pathophysiology, signs and symptoms, differential diagnosis, work-up plans, treatment choices, and expectations of outcome. They can consult millions of web pages, blogs, social media sites, podcasts, and videos in their quest for health and wellness education and support; and since all of this progress has occurred in the past 50 years, one is left to wonder what the next half century will bring.

Of course, this is also a cautionary tale. As an unregulated self-publishing platform, the Internet allows any person from any background and with any agenda to freely publish as they wish, and the individual information seeker is as likely to come across anecdotes, myths, and misconceptions as they are to uncover trustworthy medical resources rooted in evidence. This is why medical professionals must maintain a presence in every corner of the digital space, not only to create the content a global community seeks but also to guide fellow Internet users to trustworthy resources that already exist.

References

1. Sutton C. Internet began 35 years ago at UCLA with first message ever sent between two computers. UCLA Engineering, September 2004. https://web.archive.org/web/20080308120314/http://www.engineer.ucla.edu/stories/2004/Internet35.htm.
2. Banks M. Making contact with compuserve. On the way to the web: the secret history of the Internet and its founders. Apress; 2008, p. 15–24.
3. Ferrarini E. The electronic newspaper: fact or fetish. Videotex – key to the information revolution. Online Ltd; 1982, p. 45–57.
4. Newman S. Electronic newspapers. KRON. 1981. https://www.youtube.com/watch?v=5WCTn4FljUQ.
5. Emerson S. Usenet: a bulletin board for unix users. BYTE, October 1983, p. 219–236. https://archive.org/stream/byte-magazine-1983-10/1983_10_BYTE_08-10_UNIX#page/n219/mode/2up.
6. NSFNET: National Science Foundation Network. Living Internet, January 2000. https://www.livinginternet.com/i/ii_nsfnet.htm.
7. Mosaic: the first global web browser. Living Internet, January 2000. https://www.livinginternet.com/w/wi_mosaic.htm.

8. Netscape: the first commercial web browser. Living Internet, January 2000. https://www.livinginternet.com/w/wi_netscape.htm.

9. Web Browser History. Living Internet, January 2000. https://www.livinginternet.com/w/wi_browse.htm.

10. Nollinger M. America, online! WIRED, September 1995. https://www.wired.com/1995/09/aol-2/.

11. Siegler MG. How much did it cost AOL to send us those CDs in the 90s? A lot!, says save case. TechCrunch, December 2010. https://techcrunch.com/2010/12/27/aol-discs-90s/.

12. The fall of Facebook. The Atlantic, December 2014. https://www.theatlantic.com/magazine/archive/2014/12/the-fall-of-facebook/382247/.

13. WebMD Corporation announces purchase of physicians' online. WebMD Corporation, January 2004. http://investor.shareholder.com/wbmd/releasedetail.cfm?releaseid=238041.

14. Woroch GA. Turning the cables: economic and strategic analysis of cable entry into telecommunications. University of California – Berkley, February 1996. https://eml.berkeley.edu//~woroch/turncabl.pdf.

15. Zickuhr K, Smith A. Home broadband 2013. Pew Research Center, August 2013. http://www.pewinternet.org/2013/08/26/home-broadband-2013/.

16. Why we nearly McGoogled it. Metro News UK, March 2009. https://metro.co.uk/2009/03/15/why-we-nearly-mcgoogled-it-545208/.

17. Parnell BA. Search engines we have known…before Google crushed them. The Register, December 2012. https://www.theregister.co.uk/2012/12/18/search_engines_we_have_known/?page=3.

18. Clark A. How Jerry's guide to the world wide web became Yahoo. The Guardian, February 2008. https://www.theguardian.com/business/2008/feb/01/microsoft.technology.

19. Gil P. What does 'Yahoo' stand for? Lifewire, April 2012. https://www.lifewire.com/what-does-yahoo-stand-for-2483337.

20. Weinberger M. 33 photos of Google's rise from a Stanford dorm room to world domination. Business Insider Nordic, October 2016. https://nordic.businessinsider.com/google-history-in-photos-2016-10/.

21. Brin S, Page L. The anatomy of a large-scale hypertextual web search engine. Comput Netw ISDN Syst. 1998;30:107–17.

22. Hanley R. From Googol to Google. Stanford Daily, February 2003. https://web.archive.org/web/20100327141327/http://www.stanforddaily.com/2003/02/12/from-googol-to-google.

23. Kopytoff V, Frost D. For early Googlers, key word is $$$. San Francisco Chronicle, April 2004. https://web.archive.org/web/20090919030812/http://www.sfgate.com/cgi-bin/article.cgi?file=%2Fchronicle%2Farchive%2F2004%2F04%2F29%2FMNGLD6CFND34.DTL.

24. Dennison S. How much is Google worth? Go Banking Rates, July 2018. https://www.gobankingrates.com/making-money/business/how-much-is-google-worth/.

25. Rosenberg S. They shall know you through your links: Jorn Barger, filters. Say everything: how blogging began, what it's becoming, and why it matters. New York: Crown; 2009, p. 74.

26. Weblogs rack up a decade of posts. BBC News, December 2007. http://newsvote.bbc.co.uk/mpapps/pagetools/print/news.bbc.co.uk/1/hi/technology/7147728.stm.

27. Colao JJ. With 60 million websites, WordPress rules the web. So, where's the money? Forbes, September 2012. https://www.forbes.com/sites/jjcolao/2012/09/05/the-internets-mother-tongue/#38a82ac869f6.

28. Choi E. So, you wanna… learn more about medical blogs. MD Magazine, March 2007. https://www.mdmag.com/journals/mdng-primarycare/2007/apr2007/pc_learn_about_medical_blogs.

29. RSS specification history. RSS Advisory Board, June 2007. http://www.rssboard.org/rss-history.

30. Kirkpatrick D. With a little help from his friends. Vanity Fair, October 2010. https://www.vanityfair.com/culture/2010/10/sean-parker-201010?currentPage=all.

31. Jardin X. Audience with the Podfather. WIRED, May 2005. https://www.wired.com/2005/05/audience-with-the-podfather/.

32. Social media statistics & facts. Statista: The Statistics Portal. 2018. https://www.statista.com/topics/1164/social-networks/.

33. Kirkpatrick D. Social networks and the Internet. The Facebook effect. Simon & Schuster; 2010.

34. Chafkin M. How to kill a great idea. Inc., June 2007. https://www.inc.com/magazine/20070601/features-how-to-kill-a-great-idea.html.

35. Friendster is the #1 social network for adults and youth in Malaysia. Friendster, October 2008. https://web.archive.org/web/20081219023712/http://www.friendster.com/info/presscenter.php?A=pr48.

36. Rupert Murdoch comments on Fox interactive's growth. SeekingAlpha, August 2006. https://web.archive.org/web/20060819183610/http://internet.seekingalpha.com/article/15237.

37. Arrington M. Facebook no longer the second largest social network. Tech Crunch, June 2008. https://techcrunch.com/2008/06/12/facebook-no-longer-the-second-largest-social-network/.

38. Awan A. The power of LinkedIn's 500 million member community. LinkedIn Official Blog, April 2017. https://blog.linkedin.com/2017/april/24/the-power-of-linkedins-500-million-community.

39. Kaplan K. FaceMash creator survives ad board. The Harvard Crimson, November 2003. https://www.thecrimson.com/article/2003/11/19/facemash-creator-survives-ad-board-the/.

40. McGirt E. Facebook's Mark Zuckerberg: hacker. Dropout. CEO. Fast company, May 2007. https://www.fastcompany.com/59441/facebooks-mark-zuckerberg-hacker-dropout-ceo.

41. Rotham L. Happy birthday, Facebook. Time, February 2015. http://time.com/3686124/happy-birthday-facebook/.

42. Cassidy J. Me media. The New Yorker, May 2006. https://www.newyorker.com/magazine/2006/05/15/me-media.

43. Number of active users at Facebook over the years. The Associated Press, October 2012. https://finance.yahoo.com/news/number-active-users-facebook-over-years-214600186%2D%2Dfinance.html.

44. Carlson N. The real history of Twitter. Business Insider, April 2011. https://www.businessinsider.com/how-twitter-was-founded-2011-4?op=1.

45. Sarno D. Twitter creator Jack Dorsey illuminates the site's founding document. Part I. Los Angeles Times, February 2009. https://latimesblogs.latimes.com/technology/2009/02/twitter-creator.html.

46. Douglas N. Twitter blows up at SXSW conference. Gawker, March 2007. https://gawker.com/243634/twitter-blows-up-at-sxsw-conference.

47. Beaumont C. Twitter users send 50 million tweets per day. The Telegraph, February 2010. https://www.telegraph.co.uk/technology/twitter/7297541/Twitter-users-send-50-million-tweets-per-day.html.

48. 200 million tweets per day. Twitter Blog, June 2011. https://blog.twitter.com/official/en_us/a/2011/200-million-tweets-per-day.html.

49. Kim S. Twitter's IPO filing shows 215 million monthly active users. ABC News, October 2013. https://abcnews.go.com/Business/twitter-ipo-filing-reveals-500-million-tweets-day/story?id=20460493.

50. Twitter usage statistics. Internet Live Stats. 2018. http://www.internetlivestats.com/twitter-statistics/.

51. Number of monthly active Twitter users worldwide from 1st quarter 2010 to 3rd quarter 2018 (in millions). Statista: The Statistics Portal. 2018. https://www.statista.com/statistics/282087/number-of-monthly-active-twitter-users/.

52. Psion Organizer One. Bioeddie's. 1984. http://www.bioeddie.co.uk/models/psion-organiser-1.htm.

53. Hormby T. The story behind Apple's Newton. Low End Mac, August 2013. http://lowendmac.com/2013/the-story-behind-apples-newton/.

54. Sellers D. Looking back: Apple's Newton line was discontinued 18 years ago. AppleWorld Today, February 2016. https://www.appleworld.today/blog/2016/2/25/looking-back-apples-newton-line-was-discontinued-18-years-ago.

55. Niccolai J, Gohring N. A brief history of palm. PC World, April 2010. https://www.pcworld.com/article/195199/article.html.

56. Woods B. The road to BlackBerry 10: the evolution of the RIM's OS and BES. ZDNet, January 2013. https://www.zdnet.com/article/the-road-to-blackberry-10-the-evolution-of-rims-os-and-bes/.

57. Apple reinvents the phone with iPhone. Apple, January 2017. https://www.apple.com/newsroom/2007/01/09Apple-Reinvents-the-Phone-with-iPhone/.

58. Wilson M. T-Mobile G1: full details of the HTC dream android phone. Gizmodo, September 2008. https://gizmodo.com/5053264/t-mobile-g1-full-details-of-the-htc-dream-android-phone.

59. Number of smartphone users worldwide from 2014 to 2020 (in billions). Statista: The Statistics Portal. 2018. https://www.statista.com/statistics/330695/number-of-smartphone-users-worldwide/.

60. Number of apps available in leading app stores as of 3rd quarter 2018. Statista: The Statistics Portal. 2018. https://www.statista.com/statistics/276623/number-of-apps-available-in-leading-app-stores/.

Myths That Prevent Medical Professionals from Engaging

3

Michael D. Patrick

> *You can either allow social media to be helpful for you or it can be harmful. I like to let it be helpful.*
>
> —Ciara

Myth 1: People Use Websites, Not Social Media, to Find Answers Related to Health and Wellness

Traditional websites, such as WebMD, Mayo Clinic and Wikipedia, remain popular sources of healthcare information among consumers, but the use of social media to find answers to questions is on the rise. According to Pew Research Center, about 70% of Americans regularly use social media [1], and 80% of all Internet users seek answers to health-related questions online [2]. Therefore, it stands to reason that millions of people engage health and wellness content on social media sites every single day. Many find the content useful and compelling. In fact, more than 40% of all consumers admit they have made healthcare decisions based on information found in their social media feeds [3].

These numbers should not surprise us. Social media tends to be an intimate experience with relationships forged among folks who have never met in person. Friendships emerge. Trust is established. In a 2012 survey conducted by Search Engine Watch, 90% of respondents in the 18- to 24-year-old age range reported trusting medical information shared by other users on social media [4]. Another survey, conducted by Healthcare Finance, revealed 40% of people use health and wellness information discovered through social media to cope with a chronic condition, incorporate a diet or exercise plan, or select a new healthcare provider [5].

The volume of health and wellness information contained within social media is a function of user willingness to share. Just as social media relationships are personal, our health as individuals and our experience with the healthcare system are also deeply personal. Sharing these experiences and outcomes with friends and family is not only a natural by-product of relationship but sometimes cathartic. To know that others share in our trials and triumphs – and to receive support and advice from those who have traveled a similar path – can be reassuring and comforting as it affords us opportunity to participate in a common human experience.

© Springer Nature Switzerland AG 2019
D. R. Stukus et al., *Social Media for Medical Professionals*,
https://doi.org/10.1007/978-3-030-14439-5_3

A 2012 survey from PwC Health Research Institute further illustrates the degree to which social media users share health and wellness information. Forty-two percent of those surveyed reported reading health-related consumer reviews. These included opinions about specific medical providers and healthcare organizations and personal experience with over-the-counter medications, prescription drugs, and medical devices. Thirty-two percent reported reading stories about a friend or family member's healthcare journey, and 29% recalled health and wellness posts from strangers. Twenty-four percent of respondents took their engagement a step further by clicking on health-related images and videos posted by other users [6]. These numbers represent millions of Americans, and although researchers have not repeated their study, we can expect the numbers to have increased since 2012 given the growing number of Americans currently engaging on today's social media platforms.

In addition to passively reading health-related articles and reviews, social media affords users the opportunity to ask questions, provide answers and follow the back-and-forth conversations of others. Perhaps the most telling indicator of social media's influence on our collective healthcare dialogue is to simply pay attention to our own, personal social media use. How often do each of us read and share health-related stories, ask questions and provide answers with our online connections? For many of us, health and wellness are a daily part of our social media activity. For others, it is a weekly or monthly venture. If you've never participated in a health-related conversation on social media, you've come to the right place. Read on as we explore the many opportunities to engage!

Myth 2: Millennials Are the Only Generation Using Social Media

Pew Research has examined American trends in social media use since 2007. In their first report, published 1 year after Facebook and Twitter opened their doors to the public, Pew reported the largest number of social media users were young. In 2007, more than half (55%) of all Americans between the ages of 12 and 17 regularly used social media sites, with MySpace and Facebook attracting the largest number of users [7].

This finding is not a surprise because youth are typically at the frontier of cultural innovation. But it's important to remember two things: the young grow up and old habits die hard. The social media pioneers of 2007 grew into the 23- to 28-year-olds of 2018, and according to Pew, they are now more engaged with social media than they were during the teenage years, with 80% of them on Facebook and YouTube, over 50% on Snapchat and Instagram, and 35% on Twitter [1].

Pediatricians can testify to the truth of these numbers as we witness millennial parents frequently making important decisions based on information in their social media feeds. Vaccine fear, refusal, and delay is one example that not only affects the life of an individual child but can also impact an entire community as seen with recent outbreaks of pertussis and measles. The supposed benefits of homeopathic

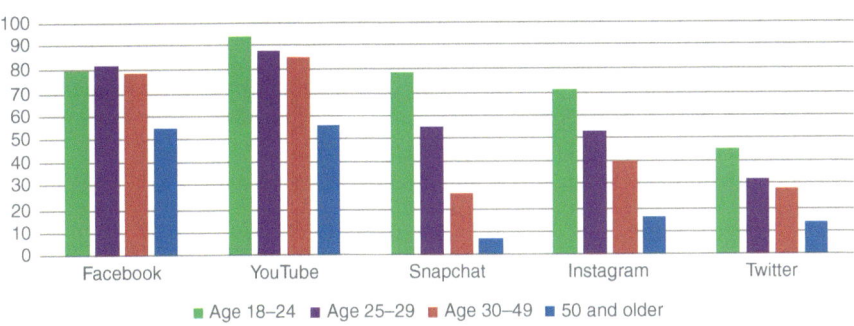

Fig. 3.1 Percentage of Americans using social media sites in 2018 by age [1]

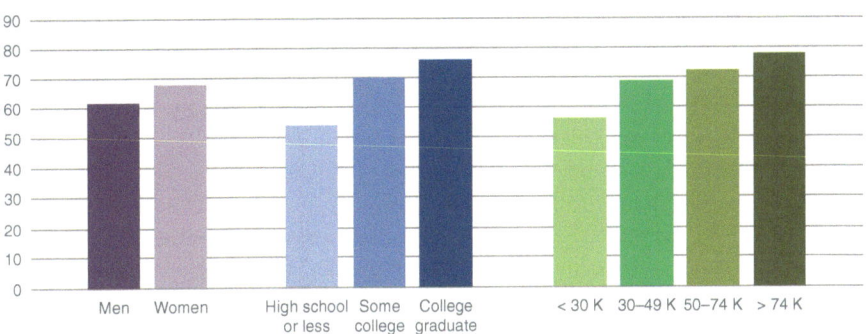

Fig. 3.2 Percentage of Americans using social media by sex, education, and income in 2015 [8]

teething products, vegetables in a pill, alternate sources of milk, and gluten-free diets are social-media-borne questions that pediatricians answer every day.

So yes, a majority of millennials use social media, and as they age, we should expect larger numbers of older Americans using these sites as a primary source of information gathering. But the truth is, in 2018, social media use by older Americans is already climbing, even among those who did not use it in previous years. Among 30- to 49-year-olds, 80% report using Facebook and YouTube, 40% use Instagram, and over 25% use Snapchat and Twitter (Figs. 3.1 and 3.2) [1].

What about older Americans in 2018 – those in the over 50 crowd who did not grow up with a computer in the home or a smartphone in the pocket? According to Pew, over half of them (55%) regularly use Facebook and YouTube. Instagram (16%), Twitter (14%), and Snapchat (7%) see less use among those over 50 [1], but as the population ages, these numbers will surely rise.

So, millennials aren't the only generation using social media, and as you think about your own practice, regardless of the age of your patients (or their parents) how often are you fielding questions brought on by something seen on social media? How often do you correct misinformation or provide an evidence-based answer to circulating fears? And what about patients and parents who don't ask questions, the ones who believe medical myths and make potentially life-altering decisions based on stories and conversations that take place online?

Rather than putting out fires after the fact, wouldn't it be better if medical professionals were in the social media trenches, answering questions based on science and pointing fellow Internet users in the direction of trustworthy resources? In this way, we could help improve the health and well-being of all Americans, regardless of their age.

Myth 3: Healthcare Consumers Don't Need My Help

We've established that millions of Americans use social media every day as they seek answers to health-related questions. Unfortunately, the answers they find are often posted by laypersons who may or may not have experienced a similar disease process. Although these posters are usually sharing in good faith, details of the disease, symptoms, diagnosis, and treatment may be inaccurate or misleading. Furthermore, those with negative experiences are more likely to take time to voice their grievances, shedding a negative spin on certain aspects of the disease or treatment process. This also provides opportunity for those with a specific agenda to misrepresent data in an effort to sway opinion.

Healthcare consumers recognize these pitfalls. Sixty percent of those seeking health information on social media say they prefer and trust posts written and shared by medical professionals [9]. This means when social media users come across differing viewpoints, they are more likely to trust us. A common example is the mother searching for information related to vaccine safety. In the course of her search, she comes across a post that warns of dangerous side effects and urges parents to skip or delay immunizations. The mom also comes across a post written or shared by a pediatrician. She learns the Vaccine Adverse Event Reporting System (VAERS) reflects associations in time rather than causation. She reads about the purpose and safety of vaccine additives, sees the exceedingly rare risks of immunizations placed alongside their many benefits, and learns the life-threatening details of vaccine-preventable diseases. The article urges her to make a decision based on evidence and reason rather than an emotional anecdote. Exposed to these differing viewpoints, most parents are apt to place greater trust in the post from the pediatrician.

Unfortunately, as we compare digital resources from medical professionals with laymen-produced content, the latter wins out in terms of sheer volume. Can we truly blame a mother's decision to delay immunizations based on her exposure to scores of anti-vaccine posts and a tiny blip from pediatric experts? At some point the greater noise wins out. The good news is that greater involvement from medical professionals will surely raise the volume of our voice, and we have plenty of room to grow. For example, nearly half of US physicians (47%) work in a practice without something as simple as a Facebook page [10]. Their patients must seek digital health information elsewhere. If patients prefer and trust online information from medical professionals, how much more would they benefit from answers obtained from the social media presence of their medical home?

So yes, healthcare consumers need our help! If they are to come across trustworthy evidence-based information in their social media feed, we have to be the ones in that space offering answers that are not only rooted in science but also readable, understandable, and useful. Sure, this takes intentional effort and skill, but as we will soon discover, a little time and practice go a long way in helping patients and families discover reliable answers that positively impact their health.

Myth 4: I'm Not Changing Anyone's Mind

Will increased social media engagement from medical professionals impact healthcare decisions and medical outcomes? This is a critical question because participation in social media takes time and effort. While one survey revealed 40% of social media users admit to making health-related decisions based on social media content [3], we do not have data on our ability to change established opinion. However, a study involving exposure to political messages on social media suggests our work can change minds.

Investigators from Lehigh University and George Mason University hypothesized that exposure to and interaction with people with differing political opinions should lead to an opinion change in some individuals [11]. They reviewed data collected from a 2012 Pew Research Center survey and identified 684 individuals who reported exposure through social media to political opinions they did not agree with. They subsequently asked these individuals two follow-up questions:

1. "Thinking about how using social networks might affect your political views overall, have you, personally, ever changed your views about a political issue after discussing it or reading posts about it on a social networking site?"
2. "Thinking about how using social networks might affect your political views overall, have you, personally, ever become more active or involved in a political issue after discussing it or reading posts about it on a social networking site?"

Seventeen percent of the respondents answered yes to the first question, and 25.5% answered yes to the second. These percentages appear small on the surface, but if the observation holds true to the general population, they represent millions of social media users whose minds have changed as a result of online exposure and discussion.

Further work by the researchers indicate people are more likely to change their minds when they are motivated and actively seeking information on a particular topic and when they are engaged with those who have a differing view. These findings support the notion that medical professionals should engage online. We should be ready to provide answers and willing to discuss the reasons for our opinions and recommendations.

But again, if our voice is missing, patients and families are less likely to hear evidence-based recommendations and guidelines and the rationale behind them. The opposing view will gain ground. We have seen this time and again in pediatrics as parents decline vaccines because of concerns over autism, neurological damage, and exposure to aluminum and mercury, despite a profound lack of evidence supporting these worries. Parents read other stories online that challenge current recommendations, including opposition to fluoride in city water supplies and promotion of infant co-sleeping. Could increased engagement with medical professionals on social media change minds regarding these important topics? The answer is a hopeful yes.

Myth 5: I'm Too Old (or Not Techy Enough) for Social Media

This misconception is plain silly. We've established that over half of seniors regularly use social media, whether medical professional or not. These numbers alone suggest old dogs can easily learn new tricks. If you report age as the primary reason for social media reluctance, please think again. What other reasons could be holding you back? Are you worried about the time commitment, not reaching a large enough audience, professional liability, or failure to gain something in return? If so, please read on and reconsider! On the other hand, if age or a perceived lack of technical know-how really is the reason, get help! It's not that difficult. Plus, it will give you a great excuse for spending a weekend afternoon with your son or granddaughter, as he or she helps you log in and shows you the ropes.

If you are an older medical professional, there is an additional reason you should engage on social media: experience! Evidence-based medicine is fantastic, but it's only as good as the studies and trials it stands upon. In many cases, the evidence is not clear. There are nuances, and not every medical case is cut from the same cloth. There are plenty of instances when recommendations change, only to revert back to the original one (think butter!). Seasoned medical professionals possess sage wisdom that can shed light on murky situations.

Here's one example. A couple of folks were recently debating vaccines on social media. One was the father of a baby girl who had passed away several years ago. Her death had come 2 days following multiple immunizations, and he was advising parents to delay or withhold vaccines because of this experience. The other was a young physician who pointed out there was no evidence to suggest the vaccines were the cause of his daughter's unexpected death. Babies die for all sorts of reasons, and just because the vaccines and death were associated in time does not mean one caused the other. The debate heated up with no signs of either side backing down or conceding a point. That is until an older pediatrician joined the conversation. She reasoned both men were arguing for the health and wellness of children. They were fighting for the same cause! Neither party changed their mind, but the view introduced by the experienced clinician extinguished the fire. Each could see the other's side with empathy, and a civil debate ensued.

Many silent onlookers followed the discourse. They learned the difference between association and causation. They learned physicians aren't taking large sums of money from Big Pharma or turning vaccine profit into family vacations. They gained insight into the motivation of many in the anti-vaccine crowd: a desire to identify a cause and prevent tragedy for another family. I imagine a few onlookers changed their view of vaccines as this conversation played out. And even though the elder physician was not a primary participant in the discussion, her wise words defused the situation and allowed thought-provoking discourse to continue.

Myth 6: Social Media Involvement Takes Too Much Time

Engagement in social media can take as little or as much time as you would like. Curating content, which is the act of gathering digital content from third-party sources to share with your social media followers, may take as little as 15 minutes a day. If you'd rather create your own content, short blog posts can be researched and written in less than 2 hours, making a weekly article quite doable with 20 minutes a day. Video posts can be made in similar fashion. Of course, if you'd like to spend more time engaging followers, curating content, or creating more time-intensive projects, such as a series of blog posts, videos, or a podcast series, have at it. Patients and families are more than eager to learn from your expertise!

After getting started, many medical professionals find themselves spending more time on social media than their schedule comfortably permits. As important as it is to engage online, it is equally important to mind our time. Family activities, working out, gardening, reading, or whatever else you like to do is immensely valuable. One strategy, aimed at providing the right amount of time each day, is the simple act of establishing a routine. Maybe it is searching for content to share in the half hour between waking up and getting out of bed. Maybe it is sitting down with a laptop at breakfast or engaging over the lunch hour. Maybe it is an hour after the kids go to bed or while (carefully) working out or taking an evening stroll. Wherever and whenever you like to spend time online, try to do it every day, and when it's time to stop… stop! It is also helpful to turn off any automatic notifications from social media to remove the constant dings or pings whenever a notification comes through – we need to be in charge of time spent on social media, not the other way around.

There are many digital tools that can save us time by automating common engagement tasks. As you collect links you'd like to share, consider placing them into a scheduling tool, such as Hoot Suite [12] or Social Jukebox [13]. In this way, you can curate in the morning, while the scheduling service posts the links to your account throughout the day. Your followers will think you are constantly thinking about them, when in practice, you are only spending that half hour over breakfast. A strategy that works for many medical professionals is to curate content for 30 minutes in the morning, schedule a few posts throughout the day and spend another 30 minutes in the evening commenting and sharing and engaging with followers.

Myth 7: Large Audiences Are Required to Make a Difference

Once you begin sharing content and interacting with other users on social media, the first statistic you are likely to watch is your number of followers. Some medical professionals have attracted extremely large audiences with tens of thousands of followers (or more!). Your followers may grow very slowly, and there may be long stretches when they do not grow at all. Sometimes they shrink. Don't be discouraged by a small following and slow growth. The work is still important. Your evidence-based information, easy-to-understand explanations, and practical tips may be the only trustworthy content your followers get. You may be the only medical professional they follow. It's a great honor that deserves your time, even when the audience remains small.

It is also important to remember that numbers of followers do not tell the whole story of our reach. Each of our followers has their own set of followers who, in turn, have their own sets of followers who, in turn, have their own sets of followers, and so it goes. By its very nature, social media is exponential. If readers find your content or commentary helpful or useful, they are likely to share. Those with whom it's shared may share, and up and out it goes, allowing your curated or original work to reach thousands of patients or families even when your particular audience is made up of less than 100 individuals.

Another point that is often overlooked is the nature of education itself. As we elevate health literacy among those online, we can expect some of our followers to alter their behaviors in life. The impact these changes have on health outcome is difficult to measure. Nonetheless, it is surely there. Impact is not only felt by those making different decisions but also their real-life social contacts as our followers share their newfound knowledge at dinner tables, daycare centers, and community groups and around the workplace water cooler. You will never know the number of lives you have changed by simply sharing and engaging with your seemingly small audience.

We should also place these "small" numbers into the perspective of a typical medical practice. The ABCs of safe sleep is an important consideration for pediatricians as they instruct parents to place babies alone, on their back, and in a crib. The average pediatrician sees about 24 patients each day. Let's say these patients are all babies, and the pediatrician shares the safe sleep message with each family. Now, this same pediatrician spends 2 hours writing a blog post about the ABCs of safe sleep. The blog post is shared on social media and ends up attracting 6000 readers in a few months' time (a reasonable possibility!). In order to impact that same number of families, our pediatrician would have to share the safe sleep message every day in every exam room for an entire year. However, social media allowed the same degree of impact with just a couple hours' work.

There's another caveat to our story. One of these 6000 readers is another pediatrician. She loves the article and shares it with her own relatively small group of followers. This eventually garners 2000 more readers. Thus, the curating pediatrician spends just 10 minutes finding, reading, and sharing the story with the equivalent impact of 4 months of daily office work.

One more consideration: even if your curated or created content is never shared by another person, even if only 1 person reads and is impacted by your work, it is still a worthwhile effort. After all, healthcare professionals have valued this degree of impact, one patient at time, in the examination room, since the dawn of medical practice.

Myth 8: Comments Are My Own; They Do Not Represent My Employer

A quick look around social media sites reveals a disclaimer in the "about me" box of many profiles: comments are my own and do not represent the views of my employer. There is a notion that this message allows the user to say anything he or she would like and provides immunity from all consequences.

This simply is not true.

High standards are required of medical professionals if we are to maintain the trust and confidence of those we serve. Messages shared on social media are essentially made to the public at large, so expect them to be read and monitored by the marketing and administrative staff of your healthcare organization. Most states in the United States view jobs as "at-will" employment, meaning an employee can quit or an employer can terminate employment at any time without warning and without establishing a just cause for the separation. In other words, you can be fired for comments made on social media, with or without a disclaimer in your profile and without your employer declaring a reason.

Another problem with a disclaimer in your profile is one of perception. Your comments may not represent the actual views of your employer, but like it or not, medical professionals are always viewed as representing their healthcare organization. We are the faces of the institution, and we always represent them in the minds of our patients and the general public. A disclaimer statement does not break the perceived association, which is why employers are very interested in what we say or do online.

Thankfully, medical professionals are allowed to share opinions. That is what we do every day in the examination room. We tell patients and families what we think, and our patients and families hold us in high regard for steering them in the right direction. Opinion-rendering translates well to the social media space as long as we continue to possess well-reasoned opinions and express them in a professional manner.

Opinions rooted in evidence work best because we can rely on science to support our views, and when science changes, we have permission to modify our opinion. When science alone fails to provide clarity, we can rely on our past experiences and form opinions based on these and any closely related data. The important thing is to explain why we think what we think and to maintain an open mind when challenged. It does not mean we will change our minds, but it is important to treat those with different viewpoints with respect (even when they do not offer us the same respect in return) and to consider and test opposing viewpoints in light of established knowledge. In other words, we should treat our encounters on social media in similar fashion to our engagement with patients and families in the clinic. This behavior, much more than a disclaimer statement, will serve to keep us in the good graces of our employers and the public because it is the behavior expected of us.

Myth 9: Social Media Engagement Is Too Risky

There are some risks associated with social media engagement. However, with a few precautions in mind, you can greatly minimize these risks and reap the many benefits of active participation.

The first precaution is to respect and maintain patient privacy. Not only is privacy a legal requirement of the Health Insurance Portability and Accountability Act of 1996 (HIPAA), it is also an important component of professional conduct. What happens in the examination room stays in the examination room. Regardless of how interesting or teachable an encounter, we must be careful to avoid details that would allow someone to identify a patient. Changing names and dates is not good enough. If you plan on sharing case studies on social media, it is best to make up details from scratch or combine events that occurred in the distant past. Never make fun of patients or criticize behavior in a derogatory way. Remember, you have not walked in your patients' shoes and are not aware of the experiences and life details that make them tick. Empathy is an important piece of professional conduct, both offline and online. Finally, if you still plan on sharing specific cases on social media, talk to someone in your institution's legal department before you post. This will ensure you have considered all possibilities and are maintaining privacy at an acceptable standard.

Never practice medicine on social media. Except for well-thought-out instances of telemedicine, there is no replacement for obtaining a face-to-face history and hands-on physical examination. Because it is nearly impossible to collect all relevant data and ensure an accurate diagnosis, the online role of the medical professional should be limited to providing educational support. We can safely answer questions about a disease process or treatment plan because we can point to the established signs and symptoms or evidence-based recommendations for treatment, but we have nothing to fall back on if we provide an incorrect diagnosis or recommend improper management for a particular patient. It is okay to answer general questions and provide helpful information, but always encourage your followers to seek the opinions and advice of their real-life medical providers.

Unless you are operating within the wheelhouse of your expertise, conduct a little research before providing comment, answering questions, or sharing content. Think about your reasons for engaging the topic and the underlying evidence that supports your opinion. Research may reveal the evidence is not as strong as you had once thought, or perhaps new evidence has come to light that changes your opinion. Not only will this ensure your comment is appropriate, but you may learn something in the process, which will benefit your office patients as well as your online followers.

Finally, think three times before you send. Once you submit a response or share content, your thoughts are out there, and you may not be able to retrieve them, even with the delete button. Shared items are difficult to erase, and screen shots capture your activity forever. However, don't let this truth keep you from participating in social media. The world needs your voice! But think about how you would reply and what you would say in mixed company. Pretend you are in an elevator or at a dinner party. Do your comments line up with how you would represent yourself in person? Avoid topics you would avoid in face-to-face professional conversations, such as certain facets of politics or religion, and enlist the help of a trusted colleague or partner to be a sounding board for comments you question sharing.

Myth 10: My Patients Won't Leave Me Alone

Social media allows real-time communication between medical professionals, patients, and the general public. Because of this ease of access, patients and providers may be tempted to use social media as a means of communication in the context of the patient-provider relationship. However, social media sites (including direct messaging features) are not secure or encrypted. Messages can be seen by others, and they can become lost in a busy feed or inbox. Consequently, social media sites are not appropriate methods of communication between providers and patients in the course of providing personal medical care. Telephone calls and secure routes of digital communication, such as the patient portal of an electronic health system (MyChart and others), continue to be the best means of sharing personal information.

Providers should clearly state this expectation to patients and families. This can occur in conversations, office policy books, signs, websites, and social media pages. Our patients should be well aware of the proper way to contact us with personal medical questions and concerns, and it is our responsibility to inform them. Of course, patients and parents will occasionally ignore this policy, but a quick and polite message of reminder can guide them back to appropriate channels of communication. With this expectation clearly set, the experience of most providers is that patients and parents appreciate engaging with their providers online regarding educational content but call or message through secure means when questions are personal and involve the health of their family.

In practice, you may find your patients contacting you less often as you engage on social media. This is particularly true as seasonal conditions emerge. Pay attention to symptoms you see and questions patients ask. These make great topics for curating, creating, and sharing with your social media followers, enabling you to anticipate questions and provide answers before patients and families have the opportunity to ask. In the world of pediatrics, a timely blog post on fever could easily prevent unnecessary phone calls and office visits. A fever post could include the reasons for fever, proper treatment, how long a typical fever lasts, and the characteristics that cause concern. It might explain fever's association with seizures and finish with a message to call the office with further questions or concerns. If you are not up for writing a blog post of your own, find one written by a colleague and share it with your followers.

Keep in mind, when your patients have questions, they will find answers. The answers they find may not be evidence-based. They may not be the answers you would have provided. By sharing the best answers online and making them available when and where your patients are looking, you can make your clinical job easier by providing reassurance and anticipatory guidance to those with questions and saving office appointments for those who truly need you.

Myth 11: I Don't Get Anything in Return

Opportunities are expanding for medical professionals to earn at least a portion of their income through social media activity and the creation of digital content. However, the vast majority of medical professionals will not generate any money from their social media presence. This is enough to dissuade many from participating. After all, medical practice is a busy endeavor, frequently involving thin profit margins and competing time interests. On the other hand, those who freely participate and count social media engagement as worthy of their time find plenty of value in the journey.

As professionals, we have a social responsibility that extends beyond our income-generating patients. The health and wellness of communities, states, and countries depend, in part, on our involvement in matters of public health and health literacy. Social media represents tremendous opportunity to impact these elements on a national (and international) scale, and the result of our collective effort serves to improve the quality of life we all enjoy.

In addition to engaging patients and the general public, social media provides a means for connecting colleagues who would not otherwise have the means to converse and collaborate throughout the year. In the distant past, these interactions took place at medical meetings or through letters and journal correspondence. The advent of email and message boards forged closer relationships among far-away peers, and social media has strengthened these bonds, allowing many to count distant colleagues as personal friends. Today, research-sharing and discussion, project collaboration, curbside consults, and the pursuit of job opportunities are all made possible through engagement on social media.

For those involved in academic medicine, social media provides a terrific opportunity to raise awareness of our work and encourage the translation of new ideas into practice. Let's face it, traditional medical journals, especially those with subscription fees, reach far fewer people than social media. Open-access peer-reviewed journals improve potential reach by paying their bills with conflict-free advertising, author fees, or grant funding. Authors can share the full text of their project through social media and invite a global community to discuss the methods, findings, and conclusion. This model of free open-access medical education serves to impact health and wellness on a grand scale, and forward-thinking academic institutions recognize the value, encourage their faculty to participate and reward their efforts with promotion.

Perhaps the most important benefit of social media participation is that digital engagement makes us better clinicians. As we connect with people online, we are

Table 3.1 Tangible benefits of social media for medical professionals	5 returns on social media investment
	1. Positive impact on health literacy and public health
	2. Keep up with changing evidence
	3. Heightened patient empathy and sharpened clinical skills
	4. Connect with distant colleagues
	5. Raised awareness of our work

forced to consider a wide range of concerns, emotions, and opinions. We find ourselves answering questions and explaining concepts we take for granted. Our clinic patients have the same questions and concerns, but these may fail to materialize in our brief face-to-face encounters. Social media engagement helps us better understand what motivates our patients and influences their decisions. It nurtures empathy and empowers us to recognize and meet previously unspoken needs and concerns in the exam room.

Additionally, as we spend time on social media sites, we are likely to come across new research that others are sharing. Large numbers of medical journals make it difficult to keep up with every new finding. However, as we follow our colleagues, we are likely to read and discuss emerging work in our field of practice. Without social media involvement, there could be significant delay in our awareness of new findings that serve to improve the health of our patients.

Finally, providing education and recommendations online motivates us to research our answers before we share them, even when we are confident the answers are correct. Of course, we also strive to provide up-to-date answers to our real-life patients, but there is a feeling of added responsibility when we post a message to the world at large. This extra step of ensuring our comments are the latest and greatest adds to our own continuing medical education. It forces us to stay current, especially in areas of active research (Table 3.1). These nimble shifts in our knowledge, based on the latest evidence and discovered through our involvement with social media, directly impact the quality of care we provide patients.

Myth 12: Other Providers Already Participate in Social Media... I'm Not Needed

Let's wrap up with a series of points we've already made, but ones particularly important and worth repeating (Table 3.2). Most people participate in social media. They trust the opinion of medical professionals. Loud voices drown out soft voices. In social media, loudness is measured by the quantity and quality of the voices in our social media feed. There are plenty of loud voices representing myths and misconceptions that negatively impact the health and wellness of our global community. The only way to counter these voices is for a multitude of medical professionals to step into the ring and speak. Nobody will do this for us, and we need every voice to make a difference, including yours!

Table 3.2 Practical steps for medical professionals to enhance their social media experience

10 steps to get you started
1. Begin with 30 minutes each day then titrate as interest and time permit
2. Stick to a schedule
3. Use an automated service, like Hootsuite, to post throughout the day
4. Respect patient privacy and maintain professionalism
5. Provide education in terms your audience can understand
6. Don't dumb down the science
7. Don't practice medicine
8. Rely on evidence and experience
9. Be practical and helpful
10. Set expectations for your patients and communicate them clearly

Conclusion

There are many barriers that prevent medical professionals from participating on social media. These include lack of time and technology skills and unfavorable perceptions of risk and profit. Healthcare professionals may feel they are unable to make a real difference or are not needed because others participate. However, with awareness and planning, these barriers can be overcome quite easily. And those who overcome them will discover many returns on their invested time, including increased empathy for patient concerns, improved communication and clinical skills, early notification of research findings, lifelong medical education, and making new connections with colleagues around the world.

References

1. Social media use in 2018. Pew Research Center, March 2018. http://www.pewinternet.org/2018/03/01/social-media-use-in-2018/.
2. Weaver J. More people search for health online. NBC News, July 2018. http://www.nbcnews.com/id/3077086/t/more-people-search-health-online/#.W-yj05NKib8.
3. 24 outstanding statistics & figures on how social media has impacted the health care industry. Referral MD, September 2013. https://getreferralmd.com/2013/09/healthcare-social-media-statistics/.
4. 33% of U.S. consumers use social media for health care info. Search Engine Watch, April 2012. https://searchenginewatch.com/sew/news/2169462/-consumers-social-media-health-care-info-survey.
5. McNickle M. 9 ways social media is impacting the business of health-care. Healthcare Finance, April 2012. https://www.healthcarefinancenews.com/news/9-ways-social-media-impacting-business-healthcare?page=1.
6. Social media 'likes' healthcare: from marketing to social business. PwC Health Research Institute. 2012. https://www.pwc.com/us/en/industries/health-industries/library/health-care-social-media.html.
7. Lenhart A, Madden M. Teens and online social networks. Pew Research Center, April 2007. http://www.pewinternet.org/2007/04/18/teens-and-online-social-networks/.
8. Perrin A. Social media usage: 2005–2015. Pew research Center, October 2015. http://www.pewinternet.org/2015/10/08/social-networking-usage-2005-2015/.

9. Infographic: healthcare industry building trust through social media. Infographics Archive. 2013. https://www.infographicsarchive.com/seo-social-media/infographic-healthcare-industry-building-trust-through-social-media/.
10. Social media & healthcare by the numbers. SMA Pulse, July 2017. https://sma.org/social-media-healthcare-by-the-numbers/.
11. Lee J, Myers T. Can social media change your mind? SNS use, cross-cutting exposure and discussion, and political view change. J Soc Media Stud. 2016;2(2):87–97.
12. Manage all your social media in one place. Hootsuite. 2018. https://hootsuite.com/.
13. Best automated social networks management tool. Social Jukebox. 2018. https://www.socialjukebox.com/.

The Role of Medical Professionals in Social Media

4

David R. Stukus

You can't believe everything you read on the internet.

—Abraham Lincoln

A Common Scenario

Every autumn, the influenza vaccine becomes available and is recommended by public health organizations and healthcare professionals. Influenza is a virus that can rapidly spread among individuals and result in severe illness, including high fever, muscle aches, and respiratory symptoms. During the 2017–2018 season, influenza caused over 30,000 hospitalizations and more than 3000 deaths in the United States [1]. Young children, the elderly, and anyone with chronic medical conditions such as cardiac problems or asthma are most susceptible to the severe effects associated with influenza. The most widely available formulation is the inactivated intramuscular vaccine, which injects proteins found in the strains of influenza most likely to cause infection that season. These proteins do not contain active virus and are incapable of causing acute infection. Common side effects from the vaccine include mild fever, soreness at the injection site, or general malaise for a day or two afterward, which is due to the normal immune response to the presence of foreign antigens. While no vaccine is 100% effective, the seasonal influenza vaccine is the best protection we can offer to help prevent infection or lessen the severity of illness.

Even in our modern healthcare system and availability of the best treatment options in the history of humanity, influenza remains a deadly virus and responsible for tremendous devastation across the world every year. Yet, despite the significant morbidity and mortality associated with influenza infection, only 37% of adults in the United States received an influenza vaccine in 2017–2018 [2]. Why is that? Vaccine refusal is a complicated topic but with the influenza vaccine, a few statements are provided as common rationale.

© Springer Nature Switzerland AG 2019
D. R. Stukus et al., *Social Media for Medical Professionals*,
https://doi.org/10.1007/978-3-030-14439-5_4

It is likely that every person reading this either knows someone who has stated or they themselves have uttered the following statement:

Every time I get the flu shot, I get the flu.

This is a common rationale offered when the influenza vaccine is deferred, along with other common reasoning tactics such as "I've never had the flu shot and I've never had the flu." So what gives? While we know that the influenza vaccine is incapable of causing anyone to develop acute infection, many people do become sick around the time they receive their vaccine. There are dozens of different viruses that circulate every autumn and winter, which can all cause various degrees of illness. Influenza vaccines are administered in healthcare facilities or public forums such as pharmacies, which are all frequented by people who are generally more likely to be sick that time of year. Any infection contracted around the time of influenza vaccine administration is coincidental and likely due to these other common exposures. In addition, many people also mistakenly self-diagnose their viral illness as "the flu," which confounds their reasoning for future vaccine avoidance. As far as those individuals who have always deferred the vaccine and have never contracted influenza, they are likely correct. Not everyone will get sick with influenza, and some will naturally experience more mild illness. However, just like the stock market, past performance is not indicative of future results.

Human nature is influenced by our many types of inherent biases which can influence anyone to naturally connect any illness, or symptoms, around the time of influenza vaccine administration with the vaccine itself. We all tend to recall the most negative or extreme examples of our past most vividly. Thus, it is natural to forget the 10 years that someone received the influenza vaccine uneventfully but focus on the 1 year they contracted a more severe illness. With social media, people can easily share these anecdotes and influence their personal networks. People who are undecided about the influenza vaccine for themselves or their children may be swayed by their friend's horrid tale of illness on Facebook. This area is ripe for alternative medicine practitioners to promote their non-evidence-based "treatments" or "natural remedies" for those wishing to avoid the pitfalls of conventional medicine. Mix a bit of pseudoscience with an ounce of personal anecdote from a convincing storyteller, and it is easy to see how this can lead to a contentious discussion in the healthcare setting.

The Power of Anecdotes

One of the challenges healthcare professionals face on social media is the need to constantly be aware of patient privacy. This will be covered in detail in Chap. 9, but in no way should any patient identifiable information be shared on social media. Professionals cannot discuss identifying characteristics of the patients they see, including gender, age, or even the date of interaction. Professionals CAN speak in general terms however (see Table 4.1 for examples). In some ways, this places

Table 4.1 Patient privacy examples for healthcare professionals who use social media

Unacceptable	Acceptable
I saw a 10-year-old boy today who had…	A common diagnosis I treat is…
My patient with Crohn's disease improved with…	Patients with Crohn's disease may benefit from…
This is a picture of a rash I saw today…	This picture depicts a rash that is frequently associated with…
Last week, a mother asked me…	A frequent question I receive from parents is…

professionals at a disadvantage on social media compared with the personal stories told by those practitioners who violate patient privacy or from patients themselves. While individuals can discuss their own health using personal and emotional stories, healthcare professionals must speak in generalities and impersonal messages. The need to honor patient privacy places healthcare professionals at a competitive disadvantage compared with the emotional stories being told by others. Personal anecdotes and testimonials are often misconstrued or viewed as evidence, or proof, of treatment efficacy. However, anecdotes often fail to capture all pertinent details pertaining to someone's care and are more likely to describe correlation, not causality.

Anecdotes can be useful in some ways, such as relaying personal stories to lead others toward evidence-based resources or to introduce a discussion on a particular topic. Media stores surrounding health-related topics often weave in an anecdote from a patient to help make the story more relatable. Anecdotes can also help raise awareness for rare or unusual situations that may not otherwise make their way into mainstream discussions. Anecdotes can also be useful in stimulating ideas leading to research of a specific diagnosis or treatment. However, anecdotes do not serve as "proof" or confirmation and can distract from scientific evidence. Potential for harm exists when anecdotes are misconstrued as evidence and important details are left out, which can impact the care of another person. In addition, false positives can occur when anecdotes falsely equate exposure with symptoms and connect two points that were present only due to correlation, not a causal relationship. False negatives can also occur when anecdotes portray lack of a connection between an exposure and harm when a causal relationship may actually exist. Needless to say, anecdotes are a dominant part of social media from the patient perspective and significantly impact how health-related information is disseminated and received.

Experienced scientists and healthcare providers versed in the scientific method understand that evidence-based medicine can rarely, if ever, "prove" anything beyond a shadow of a doubt. The nature of research is to identify factors associated with specific questions or differences between two groups. The scientific method is a trusted, reliable, systematic approach to generating and testing hypotheses but is not designed to supply absolute proof. The power of the scientific method lies in unbiased and reproducible results that support a hypothesis. This approach is foreign to many people and can be confusing, particularly since it differs greatly from other arguments or discussions. For example, trial lawyers can successfully defend their client by introducing enough conjecture and doubt to prevent the prosecutor from "proving beyond a shadow of a doubt" whether their client is guilty. Healthcare professionals are the experts called upon to defend the scientific method and can use social media to help raise awareness, introduce these difficult concepts, and discuss ways in which science can be utilized to systematically understand how our world works.

When speaking of evidence-based medicine on public forums such as social media, healthcare professionals should refrain from using medical jargon or complex terminology that is not likely understood by the lay public. It takes practice to communicate in a manner that doesn't "dumb down the science" yet present complicated information in a manner that is clearly understood. Health literacy is the degree to which individuals have the capacity to obtain, process, and understand basic health information needed to make appropriate health decisions. Unfortunately, only 12% of adults have proficient health literacy, which means almost 90% of adults lack the skills needed to manage their health and prevent disease [3]. Many of these same individuals with low health literacy will be seeking medical information online, which may lead to poor understanding or misinterpretation of available information. There are many factors that impact an individual's level of health literacy and, in turn, how that impacts their personal care (Table 4.2). Healthcare professionals must be aware of their individual patient's health literacy when discussing their care one-on-one in the healthcare setting. However, when using social media, the health literacy of an entire intended audience must be accounted for when posting medical information. Healthcare professionals who successfully engage with social media can gain valuable skills in communication which can translate to improving their communication with individual patients.

Social media grants an excellent opportunity for healthcare professionals to comment on research studies, especially when putting the findings in the proper context. Media headlines often miss the mark and overstate findings or use clever wording in an effort to generate more clicks. There are many great examples of healthcare professionals establishing a role on social media through these types of efforts.

Table 4.2 The impact of health literacy

Factors affecting an individual's health literacy	Ways low health literacy can affect individuals
Communication skills	Difficulty navigating the healthcare system, i.e., filling out forms or finding services
Knowledge base	Poor ability to communicate health history
Culture	Decreased self-management skills and impaired chronic disease management
Demands of the situation/context	Poor ability to understand concepts such as probability and risk

The anecdotes provided by patients or alternative medicine providers often describe outliers or "miracle treatments." They may originate from individuals who truly experienced an unexpected improvement in their medical condition when traditional medicine did not provide relief. Unfortunately, this is also an area where those looking to profit from misinformed patients can prosper. Even if healthcare professionals are not engaged with social media, it is beneficial to become familiar with these anecdotes to better understand why their own patients may be seeking unproven therapies or are dissatisfied with traditional medicine.

Healthcare professionals should refrain from disputing individual patient anecdotes online in social media forums. It will be extremely difficult to discuss their personal care without either violating their privacy or generating negative emotional responses. These discussions are visible to anyone and can negatively impact one's online reputation. In addition, healthcare professionals are well versed in the many nuances and specific details that pertain to an individual patient's medical care that make their personal story unique and not necessarily applicable to others. It is much more challenging to convey these thoughts on social media. However, accounts from other healthcare providers who tout non-evidence-based medicine or who are clearly attempting to profit from providing misinformation are fair game for healthcare professionals to engage with online, but these interactions should be conducted as professionally as possible. Familiarity with the Dunning-Kruger effect (Fig. 4.1) can be beneficial in these types of online interactions as those who don't receive formal education or clinical training may simply not know what they don't know. This can be confusing as they attempt to provide information commiserate with their level of training and may not be intentionally trying to provide misinformation. This is a tricky, yet important, area to navigate on social media and requires a unique skill set and experience to successfully mediate.

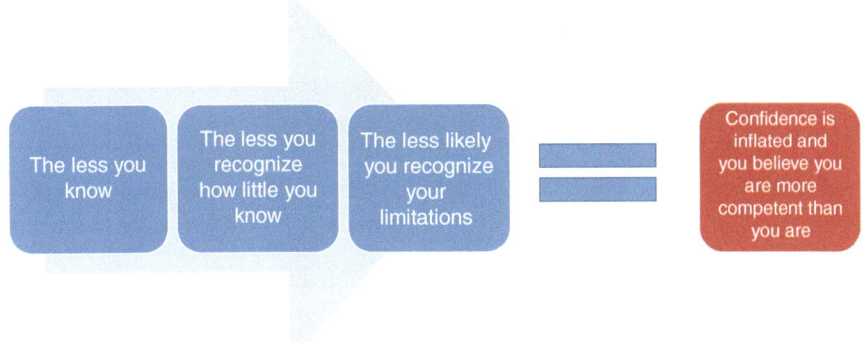

Fig. 4.1 How the Dunning-Kruger effect pertains to advice from unqualified professionals

The Quality of Evidence Matters

In our era of "fake news" and opinionated vocal personalities using social media to disseminate misinformation to advance their agendas, it is increasingly difficult for patients, the general public, and even the media to understand what constitutes high-quality evidence. Online pay-to-publish journals make it easy for any research study to find a home in a "peer-reviewed" medical journal, and it is challenging to understand how the standards these predatory journals use are much lower than trusted and respected journals with high impact factors. By cherry-picking data, misrepresenting data, and employing use of cognitive biases and pseudoscience (discussed in depth later in this chapter), seemingly valid arguments are frequently made on social media by individuals touting non-evidence-based approaches to diagnostic testing or treatment approaches. If healthcare professionals are not present on social media to disseminate evidence-based health-related information, then the information available online will not be balanced, and misinformation will prevail.

There are many factors that contribute to the quality of research studies and scientific evidence supporting a particular topic (Fig. 4.2). All too often, YouTube videos, personal anecdotes, blog posts, and websites promoting products or services are confused with evidence or given equal consideration with peer-reviewed scientific studies. Clinical guidelines employ a rigorous process through which all relevant research studies are reviewed and graded according to their methodology and findings and then combined and presented in a manner that also includes the level of evidence supporting a recommendation. Next time you read a clinical guideline,

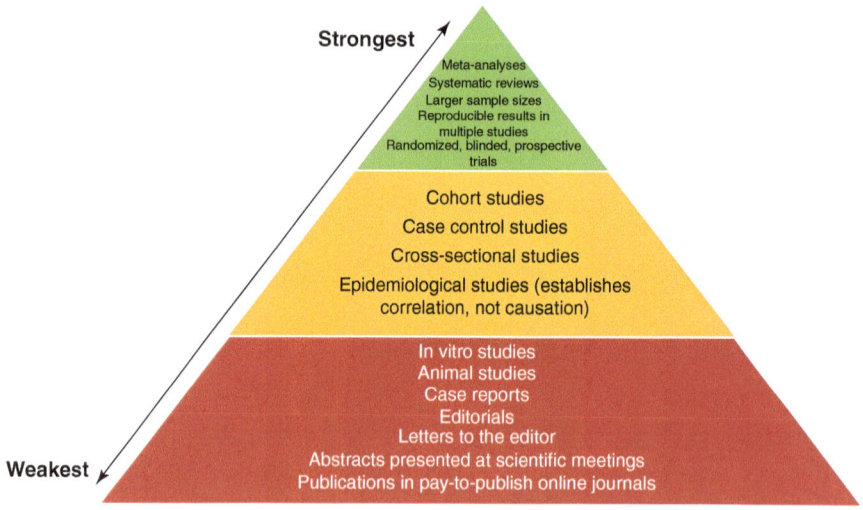

Fig. 4.2 Hierarchy of scientific evidence

pay attention to the level of evidence attributed to each recommendation. You may be surprised to learn that much of the "evidence-based" recommendations are not supported by high-quality evidence and this exercise can help increase familiarity with how guidelines are generated. Study design, sample size, outcome measure, type of intervention, inclusion/exclusion criteria, randomization, study duration, and statistical analyses are just some of the important details that determine the quality of a study and its findings. Healthcare professionals and researchers spend years learning how to interpret research studies and even then often fail to recognize and appreciate study limitations. With more open-access journals and public access to entire research studies, anyone can read the same study, but if they lack the appropriate training, education, and experience, then findings can easily be misinterpreted and overgeneralized.

One way healthcare professionals can use social media is to highlight flawed interpretation of study findings from media reports or online discussions. This is an area where the general public generally appreciates our voice and expertise. Most professional and patient advocacy organizations that disseminate research findings or media reports have a team of medical experts that read, interpret, and assist in the messaging utilized on their public facing social media platforms and website. However, the rise in bloggers who focus on specific health conditions has led to a virtual army of individuals who often have the best intentions but report every research study related to their interest either misinterpretation or lack of interpretation and often without appropriate context to help readers best understand how the information applies to their own health. This is where healthcare professionals can have a helpful presence on social media, either in understanding the application of specific research findings, or in discussing the overall approach to understanding the hierarchy of evidence.

This may come as a shock, but 59% of links shared on Twitter ARE NEVER EVEN READ BY THE PERSON SHARING THEM! [4]. People are receiving their information from simply reading the headline alone. Thus, media reports and catchy headlines that misinterpret, overstate, or confuse research findings can easily be misinterpreted by many individuals on social media. To understand the scope of this, you can set a Google alert for articles related to any topic of interest to receive a vast array of examples, or you can search online for media stories pertaining to a specific topic. Spend some time paying attention to the headlines media outlets used to generate clicks and shares, *then* read the article, and *then* locate and read the actual research study. More often than not, you will find that the information provided in the article is either missing the mark in regard to overall study findings or cherry-picked one particular aspect that was deemed more popular or likely to generate interest while ignoring important study limitations or additional findings. For healthcare professionals engaging in social media, it is important to understand this common behavior not only in how people discuss information but for how they formulate their own decisions. In addition, healthcare professionals can take advantage of this aspect to generate interest in their own posts and increase their audience. See a few examples of my approach in Fig. 4.3.

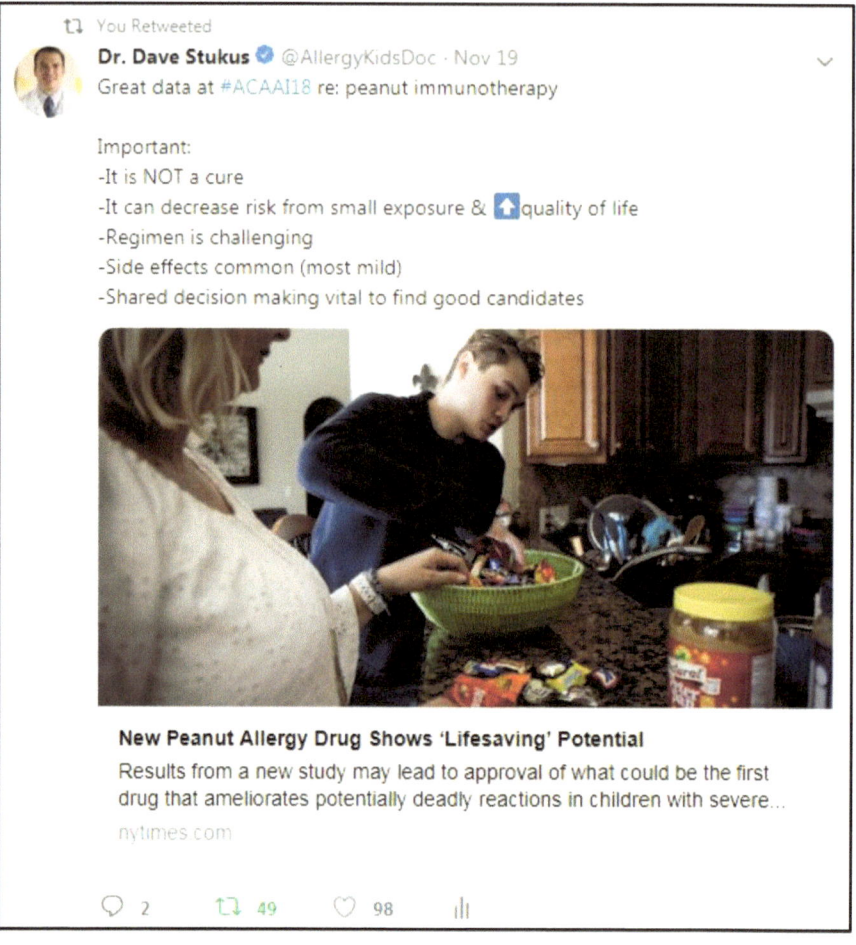

Fig. 4.3 Providing comments on media reports can help clarify misrepresentation of study findings. (Adapted from https://twitter.com/AllergyKidsDoc)

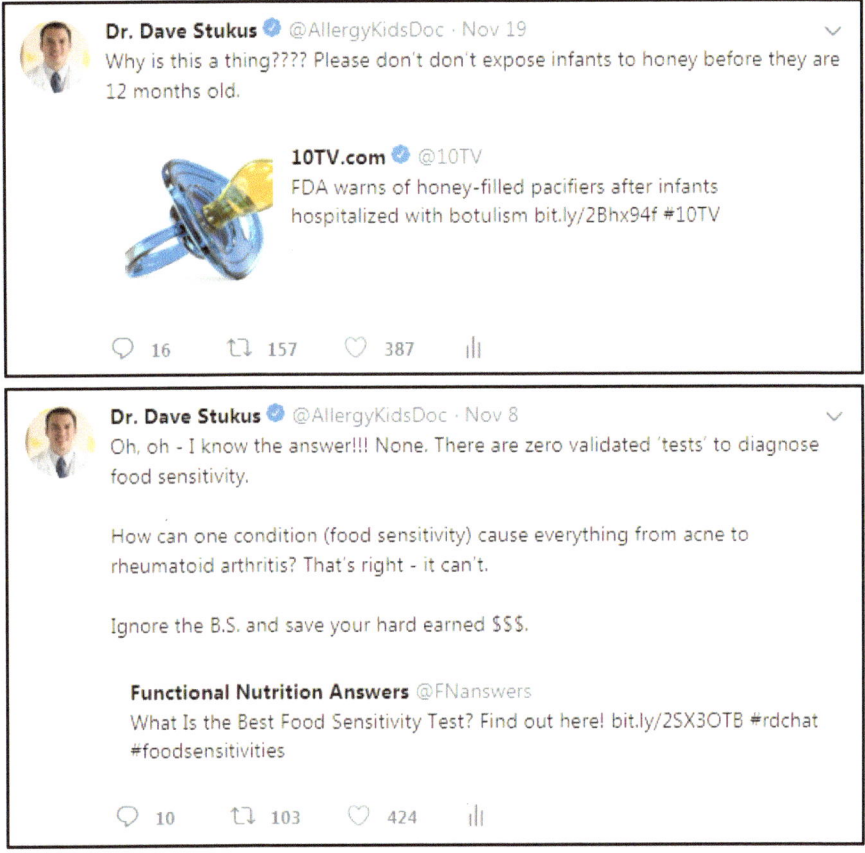

Fig. 4.3 (continued)

The Echo Chamber Effect

The circulation of bad advice, poor-quality evidence, and articles that are never read past the headlines within social media circles leads to an echo chamber effect. Users are more likely to share headlines or stories that align with their pre-existing opinions and beliefs. Likewise, information that challenges their beliefs are less likely to be circulated. As a result, publishers will focus their headlines and stories on those that will generate the most interest and clicks. For example, rare examples of stories surrounding airline passengers with peanut allergy who do not receive certain accommodations or who report allergic reactions in flight receive much more attention than the reality of thousands of people with peanut allergy flying safely every month. A headline such as "Thousands of airline passengers with peanut allergy arrived to their destination with no symptoms or concerns" is not nearly as emotional or click worthy as "Passenger with peanut allergy had severe reaction after airline refused to stop serving nuts." Social media groups then regurgitate the same types of posts and content, which leads to confirmation bias, lack of thoughtful consideration of other viewpoints, and information stagnation.

Cognitive Bias

We all have cognitive biases, which are systematic patterns that deviate from the norm and interfere with our ability to make rational decisions [5]. This section will highlight many examples of cognitive biases which commonly occur within ourselves, our patients, and are rampant online. Healthcare professionals who have a thorough understanding of cognitive biases and how they can dramatically impact one's perception of reality will easily recognize these throughout social media. This can help not only better understand online behavior, but can also offer a unique advantage in online interactions. In other words, if we can understand and identify the common faults in how people make decisions related to their health, we can point these out, provide a rational explanation, and ideally realign their decision-making. *This may be our secret weapon in navigating social media as healthcare professionals.*

Cognitive biases lead people to create their own personal subjective reality, which can dictate behavior. As you can imagine, if everyone is viewing the world according to their own perception, this can lead to false conclusions that lie well outside proven facts, science, and reality. A striking example of this concept was highlighted in a 2018 survey conducted by YouGov that showed 2% of Americans believe the world is flat [6]. You may want to read that sentence again and let that sink in for a moment: Two percent of Americans believe our planet is flat. Among the respondents to this survey who were 18–24 years old, 4% of them believed the world is flat and only 66% were "sure" that the world is round.

Social media is an online community with billions of individual users, each connected with one another in real time and with the freedom to disseminate any information they choose and comment on posts by any other user. It behooves healthcare professionals to appreciate the wide range of viewpoints, biases, and alternate perceptions of reality that members of their audience possess. Ultimately, we should all expect the unexpected and become comfortable walking away from any interactions that cause us to want to bang our head against the wall, so to speak.

The following is a list of cognitive biases that can impact decision-making regarding health conditions. Once you are familiar with this list, it will be helpful to spend time on various social media platforms to identify examples of each. With time and practice, it will be difficult to *not* see these various examples, which are exceedingly common online.

- *Aggregate bias* – A belief that aggregated data, such as those used to develop clinical guidelines, do not apply to individual patients. A belief that an individual is atypical or exceptional may lead to unnecessary testing or treatment when guidelines indicate none are required.

- *Ambiguity effect* – Avoidance of options when the probability is unknown. This leads to a tendency to consider a diagnosis for which a probability of treatment outcome is known over one that is unknown.
- *Bandwagon effect* – The tendency for people to believe and do certain things because many others are doing so. See: gluten-free diets, the billion dollar supplement and vitamin industry, widespread use of essential oils, etc.
- *Base-rate neglect* – Ignoring the true prevalence of a disease, either through inflating or reducing its base rate. This distorts the perception of a certain diagnosis likely to be present.
- *Belief bias* – The tendency to accept or reject data depending upon one's personal belief system. Examples include rejection of the HPV vaccine to prevent a sexually transmitted virus that causes cancer due to the belief that this will promote promiscuity among teenage recipients. See also: climate change denialism based upon political belief systems.
- *Confirmation bias* – The tendency to seek confirming evidence to support a diagnosis or argument rather than look for disconfirming evidence to refute it. This leads to ignoring evidence that refutes previously held beliefs and giving less credible information more weight if it supports previously held beliefs. *Confirmation bias is rampant among individuals who have done their own "research" surrounding a health condition by using online search engines.*
- *Framing effect* – The manner in which a history is provided can strongly influence decision-making. Patients may emphasize certain aspects or symptoms they deem more important while ignoring other meaningful aspects of their history.
- *Hawthorne effect* – The tendency for people to behave differently (usually making themselves look better than they really are) when they know they are being observed. This is social media at its essence. Very few people will discuss their personal downsides on social media, which in effect creates an online community where everyone is presenting their best version of themselves for the world to see.
- *Illusory correlation* – Falsely attributing correlation with causality. This is a common error when findings from research studies not designed to investigate a causal relationship are used to support non-evidence-based approaches to health.
- *Personal example: For unknown reasons, rates of food allergies have increased over the past two decades. Various "causes" have been touted by some with ulterior motives, including those who oppose vaccines and genetically modified organisms, despite no evidence supporting any causal relationship. I like to use this rebuttal to highlight the important difference of correlation with causality. "It is an undeniable FACT that rates of food allergy have doubled since [popstar] Justin Bieber was born." While this is a true statement, no one can rightfully blame Justin Bieber for causing the rise in food allergies.
- *Information bias* – The tendency to believe that the more evidence one can accumulate to support a decision, the better. Unfortunately, this lends itself to using poor-quality evidence or making connections that don't exist in formulating a decision.

- *Omission bias* – The tendency toward inaction. In hindsight, events that have occurred through natural disease progression are more acceptable than those that may be attributed directly to action of the healthcare professional. For example, a story of someone who died from cancer while receiving unproven alternative treatment is viewed more favorably than someone who died of cancer while receiving chemotherapy but suffering from side effects.
- *Overconfidence bias* – This is a universal tendency to believe we know more than we do, which is pervasive and powerful. Opinions are given more weight than quality evidence. This is a significant challenge for healthcare professionals who engage in social media – despite their experience, training, and expertise, online platforms and overconfidence bias diminish their contributions and overweigh the opinions of patients and lay people.
- *Self-serving bias* – The tendency to claim more responsibility for successes than failures. This bias is present throughout social media from alternative medicine practitioners who tout miracle "cures" or 100% success from their approach, particularly when doing so in the name of making a profit from their supplements, books, or services.

Heuristics

A heuristic technique, or heuristic, is any approach to problem-solving, learning, or discovery that employs a practical method, which is not necessarily logical or rational, that is sufficient for reaching an immediate goal [7]. Heuristics are very similar to cognitive biases and can be thought of as shortcuts people use to solve problems and make judgments quickly and efficiently (Table 4.3). Heuristics can lead to the development of biases by introducing errors in judgment regarding how common things occur and how representative certain things may be.

There are a few common heuristics that people use in making decisions pertaining to their health:

Table 4.3 Examples that employ heuristics

Heuristic	Definition
Rule of thumb	Not intended to be strictly reliable in every situation; based on practical experience
Educated guess	Using one's experiences and knowledge of similar situations to make an initial guess, which can be confirmed or denied later
Intuition	Knowledge without proof, evidence, conscious reasoning, or understanding of how the knowledge was acquired
Guesstimate	An estimate derived from incomplete information
Stereotyping	Judging a group different from one's self based upon opinion or prior encounters
Profiling	Using personal characteristics or behavior patterns to make generalizations about a person
Common sense	Sound practical judgment when encountering everyday matters

- *Availability heuristic* – People overestimate the importance of information that is available to them. For instance, a person might argue that smoking is not unhealthy because they know someone who lived to be 100 years old and smoked three packs a day. Or someone with peanut allergy suddenly feels they are no longer safe in public spaces after reading a tragic story of someone dying from accidental ingestion of peanut, even though they have safely been in public areas for years without any problems.
- *Representativeness heuristic* – Making a decision by comparing the present situation to the most representative mental prototype. Imagine trying to decide if someone is trustworthy. If they are an older person who reminds you of your grandmother, their traits may line up with your mental prototype of a gentle and trustworthy individual.
- *Affect heuristic* – Making choices strongly influenced by emotions experienced at that moment. Mood can impact decisions regarding risk and benefit, i.e., someone with asthma feeling that they'll never be able to play sports when presented with information, while they are feeling upset or angry about a situation.
- *Anchoring* – The human tendency to rely more heavily on the first piece of information offered (the "anchor") when making decisions. For example, a person may lock on to salient features of their initial presentation and fail to adjust their initial impression despite new symptoms or changes in their health.
- *Escalation of commitment* – People justify increased investment in a decision based upon cumulative investment, despite new evidence suggesting that the cost, starting today, of continuing the decision outweighs the benefit. This is common with financial investments. Imagine investing $10,000 into stock for a promising and widely discussed company in 2008. Due to various problems with the company's production facilities and public relations, the stock slowly and gradually declines in value, and by 2018 the initial investment is now only worth $5000. The data indicate no reason to continue with this investment and the money should be reallocated to invest in other ventures. However, due to the longstanding commitment and initial promise of returns, people are more likely to hold on to their initial investment, essentially doubling down on their own money and time even with certain losses in their future.

Pseudoscience 101

The boundary between science and pseudoscience is often murky. Pseudoscience basically consists of statements, beliefs, or practices that are claimed to be both scientific and factual, but are incompatible with the scientific method. Social media is the perfect platform for attention grabbing headlines and pseudoscientific explanations for unproven diagnostic testing or treatment options to gain traction and widespread appeal. Think of every headline you've read regarding cellphones causing cancer, the hidden power of detoxes and cleanses, or how gluten is ravaging our bodies – that is pseudoscience 101. Why does the public fall for this…often to the point of spending large amounts of money for treatment options or programs that are not supported by any evidence? Our cognitive biases contribute, but another phenomenon may be contributing to this as well.

Traditionally, science has been communicated to the public by those in academics, who, to the average person, may seem elitist, nerdy, or disconnected. As discussed elsewhere throughout this textbook, scientists and healthcare professionals have generally missed the mark when trying to communicate health-related information to the general public. However, as also mentioned, we know that people are searching online for health-related information. As such, this space has been filled by professionals who overreach their qualifications, such as chiropractors, homeopaths, naturopaths, and other alternative medicine providers (plus the occasional board-certified physician who has crossed over to the dark side of pedaling pseudoscience in the name of profit). These individuals have traditionally excelled at communicating and listening to patients, which in turn, makes them more seem more trustworthy and believable. While some of these individuals deliberately dispense misinformation in an attempt to profit from their services, many are subject to the Dunning-Kruger effect and are merely explaining things in a way they were taught in their alternative medicine education. They simply don't know what they don't know and fill in the gaps with thought processes that are often not physiologically plausible and rarely supported by evidence. Regardless of intent, this is an important arena that contributes to the vast array of misinformation online, confuses patients and the public, and by muddying the waters, ultimately leads to decreased trust in qualified healthcare professionals who are dispensing evidence-based information.

Unfortunately, modern medicine has failed to find a cure, and in some cases effective treatment, for many chronic conditions. Patients can easily become frustrated when healthcare professionals dismiss their chronic ailments and concerns or fail to provide any relief. It is only natural for them to turn to unproven therapies in the quest to find relief from their struggles. This is where they can be taken advantage of through promises of magical cures or providers who claim to know the "cause" of their complaints (occasionally with disparaging remarks about how medical schools don't teach the "right" information). Chronic Lyme disease, chelation therapy, vaccine toxicity, toxic mold syndrome, electromagnetic sensitivity, and bogus cancer treatments are just a few areas where pseudoscience prevails. Harm occurs when patients forego proven evidence-based treatment options in favor of unproven therapies, spend significant amounts of money, and experience side effects, at times severe, from pursuing this path. This is one of the most profound reasons why healthcare professionals should disseminate evidence-based information through social media: to try to reach some of these patients and prevent their descent into the realm of pseudoscience.

Use of specific wording (Fig. 4.4), conspiracy-fueled rejection of evidence-based recommendations, and cherry-picked data from research studies performed in laboratory animals or presented as abstracts at scientific meetings but not published in peer-reviewed journals are a few tactics used by those peddling

Inflammation	Free radicals	Detox	Celebrity endorsement	Energy
Cleanse	Fatigue	Crystals	Naturopathic	All natural
Chemical free	Ancient Wisdom	FREE SPACE	Instinctively know best	Organic
Conspiracy	Molecules	Toxins	Cure	'Western' Medicine
Pharma shills	"Science doesn't know everything"	Government/ mind control	Miracle	Magnetic

Fig. 4.4 Pseudoscientific bingo – common words and phrases used to provide exaggerated claims

Table 4.4 How to spot pseudoscience by answering a few simple questions. Answer choices with the "X" should raise red flags regarding credibility

Question	Yes	No
Does the claim come from a reputable resource?		X
Does the claim rely entirely on testimonials?	X	
Does the claim promise a secret or truth that was "intentionally" withheld until now, i.e., conspiracy theory?	X	
Is the health issue likely to resolve without treatment?	X	
Is there a clinical trial or peer-reviewed study that supports the claim?		X
Have similar results been replicated with other studies?		X
Is there any evidence to support the claim?		X

pseudoscience. Healthcare professionals can assist patients and the public in identifying and avoiding pseudoscience by promoting positive messaging on social media and raising awareness. Timothy Caulfield, who wrote the book *Is Gwyneth Paltrow Wrong About Everything: When Celebrity Culture and Science Clash*, and Jennifer Gunter, an obstetrician/gynecologist, are prominent examples of healthcare professionals who have used social media to combat pseudoscience, disseminate evidence-based information, and generate large followings. Their blend of humor, sarcasm, and, most importantly, clear explanations of complicated medical information are mainstays to their successful approach. They, along with others, fight back against pseudoscience using similar tactics to those peddling woo… fighting fire with fire, so to speak.

A series of simple questions can be asked about every article or website to help determine whether the powers of pseudoscience may be at work (Table 4.4).

Why Healthcare Professionals NEED to Be Engaged in Social Media

We know that patients are going online to find health information. By using common search engines, they can easily encounter websites and social media accounts that provide misinformation which distracts from proper diagnosis or treatment. Anecdotes, cognitive biases, and pseudoscientific explanations are common themes that contribute to these challenges. If healthcare professionals are not claiming this space and providing evidence-based information, then misinformation prevails.

A responsibility that healthcare professionals who use social media should take seriously is the need to provide evidence-based information and use vetted resources. However, it is still acceptable to offer an opinion based upon experience and clinical expertise but it should be clarified when this occurs. Including links to published research studies, clinical guidelines, or professional organizations will provide a vetted resource for followers and members of the target audience to read for additional information. Social media has limitations in regard to length of posts or types of information provided; thus inclusion of links to longer articles or references can be a very helpful addition. A bonus to this approach is the learning that can occur BY the healthcare professional, whose knowledge base and understanding of the evidence can grow through online interactions and through the process involved in posting vetted medical information.

There are many ways in which professionals can engage with social media, which will be explored in greater detail through the next several chapters. It can be overwhelming at first, and it can be useful to start slow, watch, and learn at the beginning. Professional organizations, academic hospital systems, and professionals from every discipline are already engaged in social media and provide excellent examples to learn some best practices. There are professional accounts across every specialty and professional background to help generate ideas and provide a good starting point. By reading this textbook, you have already demonstrated an interest in this realm, which distinguishes you from your colleagues not engaged in social media. Now it's time to take some first steps or, for those already active, employ some new strategies, to grow your online presence and create a large platform. Norman Rockwell created iconic paintings and lasting images of physicians depicted as distinguished and respected professionals engaging with one patient at a time. For better or worse, those days are long gone, and physicians and healthcare professionals need to adapt to how the rest of the world communicates, disseminates information, and engages in real time across networks that span the globe. While healthcare professionals treat one patient at a time in clinical encounters, they can now grow a large online platform enabling them to reach thousands of patients. Considering that use of social media has little financial cost associated with it, other than one's time commitment, the value is tremendous…even if only one patient ever reads a post.

Healthcare professionals who use social media can benefit in many ways other than the dissemination of evidence-based information and interactions with the general public [8]. They can join online communities to read news articles, interact with experts in their field, stay abreast of medical and research developments, consult colleagues regarding patient issues (only through secure formats or by following patient privacy laws) and network with colleagues from across the world. Personally, I have engaged in social media in all of these ways and have virtually "met" many colleagues from across the world online and formed professional relationships that have translated to various collaborative efforts. In addition, social media can help professionals disseminate their own research findings and ideas, discuss practice management strategies, market their practices, and engage in health advocacy.

As discussed in Chap. 1, not all social media platforms are ideal for purposes of healthcare professionals engaging with social media. The risk of spreading one's self too thin across multiple platforms must also be considered, not only in regard to time management but in diluting the messages as well. It's always best practice to focus on what you know and can do well first, and then you can experiment with extending your reach.

I'm a Doctor on Social Media, but I'm Not YOUR Doctor

Healthcare professionals who develop a large platform through social media will increase their visibility and accessibility. As such, patients and the general public will likely start to engage more and ask for specific medical advice regarding their personal care. Healthcare professionals should NEVER offer specific medical advice through social media, even through direct messages or more secure channels hidden from the public. There are too many nuances to one's personal history that cannot be conveyed through social media and can impact a diagnosis or treatment suggestions. In addition, a physical examination cannot take place, and important details pertaining to comorbid conditions, family history, and confounding factors are neglected. Healthcare professionals who do offer individual medical advice can be held liable if their advice is incorrect or leads to harm. It is important for everyone to be aware of this downside and also prepare for the inevitable questions they may receive.

It can be useful to have standard, responses drafted and ready to use in these circumstances. It is always helpful to direct patients to their own personal provider or vetted sources of general information pertaining to their condition or line of questioning. A standard reply that I have adopted has been very useful:

> Thank you for reaching out. Unfortunately, I am unable to provide any individual medical advice through social media. I encourage you to contact your personal physician with your questions, as they are best equipped to offer specific advice pertaining to your individual care. Thank you for understanding and best wishes.

I receive many requests for personal advice through my Twitter feed, sometimes as often as daily, and this standard approach is always well received. Patients understand when I point out my limitations and I have yet to receive any confrontational replies. In addition, I have also been proactive with my own patients who use social media, and I inform them that they should not contact me online for any specific questions or to discuss personal information. I also inform them that I cannot acknowledge that I know them, like their comments, friend them, or indicate that they are my patient as a manner of protecting their privacy…not to be rude. As our relationships with patients evolve, it will serve us all well to keep their best interests in mind.

Conclusion

Healthcare professionals can personally benefit in many ways by engaging online through social media. More importantly, we can serve as credible sources of evidence-based information and provide a vetted landing spot for those seeking health information online. It is useful to understand the array of misinformation available online, including origins, and ways to combat it. Through our understanding of cognitive biases and pseudoscience, we can address these aspects through our approach on social media and our attempts to provide a guided path.

References

1. Summary of the 2017–2018 influenza season, Centers for Disease Control. https://www.cdc.gov/flu/about/season/flu-season-2017-2018.htm. Accessed 13 Dec 2018.
2. Estimates of influenza vaccination coverage among adults—United States, 2017–18 flu season, Centers for Disease Control. https://www.cdc.gov/flu/fluvaxview/coverage-1718estimates.htm. Accessed 13 Dec 2018.
3. Kirsch IS, Jungeblut A, Jenkins L, Kolstad A. Adult literacy in America: a first look at the results of the National Adult Literacy Survey (NALS). Washington, DC: National Center for Education Statistics, U.S. Department of Education; 1993.
4. Gabielkov M, Ramachandran A, Chaintreau A, Legout A. Social clicks: what and who gets read on Twitter? ACM SIGMETRICS/IFIP Performance 2016, June 2016, Antibes Juan-les-Pins, France. 2016. <hal-01281190>.
5. Norman GR, Monteiro SD, Sherbino J, Ilgen JS, Schmidt HG, Mamede S. The causes of errors in clinical reasoning: cognitive biases, knowledge deficits, and dual process thinking. Acad Med. 2017;92(1):23–30.
6. https://today.yougov.com/topics/philosophy/articles-reports/2018/04/02/most-flat-earthers-consider-themselves-religious. Accessed 13 Dec 2018.
7. Blumenthal-Barby JS, Krieger H. Cognitive biases and heuristics in medical decision making: a critical review using a systematic search strategy. Med Decis Mak. 2015;35(4):539–57.
8. Venola CL. Social media and health care professionals: benefits, risks, and best practices. P T. 2014;39(7):491–9.

The Art of Digital Storytelling

5

Michael D. Patrick

> *I would rather entertain and hope that people learned*
> *something than educate people and hope they were entertained.*
>
> —Walt Disney

Why We Should Become Storytellers

Walt Disney recognized the value of adding educational elements to his entertainment projects. Likewise, we can add effectiveness to our teaching when we weave it into an entertaining framework. Think about your favorite teachers and speakers. Do they present monotone presentations riddled with difficult-to-read graphs and dozens of bullet points, or are they dynamic, engaging storytellers? Think too about your web browsing and social media habits. Unless we are highly motivated for a specific data point, most of us spend more time with content, ponder its meaning, and incorporate the information into our knowledge base, when it is meaningful and presented in an engaging way. What about content we abandon as we explore the web and our social media feeds? What happens when the content creator fails to reel us in? How long do we tolerate information that lacks relevance and benefit to our lives? How long do we linger on boring content before moving on to something else? The truth is if when we fail to engage, our teaching falls flat, our audience loses interest, and our mission of improving health and wellness fails.

So how can we engage our audience? How can we teach and entertain? One method is to present our content as a story. Stories provide more than basic facts. They explain what something is, how it works, and why it is relevant. Stories build connections and empower people to put knowledge into action. Newspaper columns and self-help magazines have shared information through stories for decades. Readers not only benefit from new knowledge, they keep coming back. Why?

© Springer Nature Switzerland AG 2019
D. R. Stukus et al., *Social Media for Medical Professionals*,
https://doi.org/10.1007/978-3-030-14439-5_5

Because stories invite us to engage. They encourage us to assimilate new information with past knowledge and experience. Most importantly, this process has the power to transform our opinions and behaviors.

Those who perpetuate medical myths are often good storytellers. They draw their audience in, trigger an emotional reaction, and present a call to action. The anti-vaccine movement is built upon personal stories and evidence that appears compelling. Tragic stories of children who exhibit new symptoms after a vaccine trigger a response that make the message matter, even though there is no evidence that one event caused the other. The subsequent call to action – to delay or forego vaccines – is strong, and many parents heed that call. How can we expect to change hearts and minds when we counter this argument with dry bullet points presented with an antagonistic tone? In order to make a difference, we too must become passionate storytellers.

So, how does one tell an effective story? First and foremost, we must connect with our audience. Those opposed to vaccines love their kids. They believe vaccines harm children, so it makes sense they would write and act with passionate opposition. Parents connect with that sentiment. They get it. We do well to understand the concern and express empathy for the anti-vaccine position. But then, we must demonstrate greater passion for the evidence because we too care about kids. There are many elements we can incorporate into an engaging pro-vaccine story. We can relate the experiences of families hurt by vaccine-preventable diseases; explain immune responses in an interesting way; connect immune responses to anticipated post-vaccine symptoms; explore the reasons and safety of vaccine additives such as mercury, aluminum, and formaldehyde; share insights from the Vaccine Adverse Events Reporting System; and place benefits and risks in their proper perspective. We can easily use these ideas to build a compelling story. We don't need to use every element every time, but we must move beyond "I'm a doctor so you should trust my opinion that vaccines are good." We may not change the minds of those solidly opposed to vaccines, but many undecided parents are watching. They consume stories from both camps, and in order for our stories to matter, we must connect and care, explain, and be helpful.

What form should medical stories take? There isn't a one-size-fits-all answer to this question, and the first idea that comes to mind may not be the best one. For example, many tell their story with lots of words, and while this format can certainly work, there are other options to choose from. Content creators can divide lengthy pieces into a series of shorter posts. An infographic can tell a story, as can podcasts, videos, and a series of tweets. We do not even need to create our own content. Curating material from other authors and strategically sharing it through social media is another effective way to tell a story.

Regardless of the form our story takes, it needs a place to start. How do we choose a topic, collect our thoughts, and determine what we want to say and how we want to say it? These questions have vexed writers for ages. It turns out, few writers sit in front of a blank page and craft a complete story in one take. The storytelling process requires intentional planning to pull off well. There are many tools writers can use to develop a story. One such method incorporates the "reporter questions" into the storytelling process.

Introducing the Reporter Questions

There are six questions every reporter asks as they frame a news story: who, what, when, where, why, and how. There are a couple ways we can use these questions in medical storytelling. First, they represent a checklist to ensure we cover our topic in a comprehensive fashion. Consider a medical story about asthma. Considering the reporter questions is important because when people search for answers on a given topic, the answer one person seeks may be different than the answer another one seeks. By including several answers, we help the largest number of people. Covering multiple aspects of asthma is also important because it paints a full picture of the disease, one that beckons audience members in with an answer to their question and then empowers them with greater understanding by weaving the answer into the bigger story.

Let's keep thinking about asthma. How can we use the reporter questions to brainstorm a framework for our story? What questions could we attempt to answer? We don't have to answer every question we conceive, but intentionally thinking about each reporter question will certainly help us build a richer story. Here are examples of potential questions:

Who is affected by asthma? Who is at risk? Who treats the disease? Who ends up in the hospital? What is asthma? What causes it? What symptoms result? When do we see these symptoms – what time of year and in what situations? What are rescue inhalers? When are they used? When should patients with asthma seek help, and where should they go – to the medical home or an urgent care center or an emergency department? Why does the place of care matter? What are steroids, why are they important, and when are they used? Why do some people have mild asthma symptoms, while others have severe problems? How does each type of asthma medication work, and how can we prevent asthma flare-ups from happening in the first place?

There are plenty more who, what, when, where, why, and how questions we could ask and answer about asthma. The point is not to include every possible question and answer, but to at least consider all of them as we choose a framework for our story. Without a broad view of the choices, it's easy to overlook an important piece of information that might help connect the dots for those seeking answers. Now think about a common topic of interest in your scope of care. Make a list of the who, what, when, where, why, and how questions for your topic, and take the first steps of framing an educational story for your patients (Table 5.1).

Table 5.1 Correlating reporter questions with health-related information

Elements of disease explained by the reporter questions	
Disease element	Reporter questions
Definition	What?
Epidemiology	Who?
Pathophysiology	When? Where? How?
Symptoms	When? Where? Why?
Differential diagnosis	What?
Work-up	Who? What? When? Where?
Treatment	Who? When? Where? Why? How?
Complications	What? When? Why?
Prevention	How?
Prognosis	Who? What?

In addition to helping us build a comprehensive story on a particular topic, the reporter questions are useful on a grander storytelling scale. We can use them to organize our thoughts and strategy as we consider WHAT we want people to know, WHY we want them to know, WHO we want to tell, HOW we want to tell it, and WHEN and WHERE to share our story.

What Do We Want People to Know?

Choosing the right topic is an important first step, and one many find difficult. We want to be relevant and helpful without adding to the massive amount of digital background noise our followers sift through every day. A good place to start is with our clinical passions. These are the items about which we are most knowledgeable and up-to-date. We emphasize them in our practice and spend more time answering patient questions and explaining how things work because these are the topics that interest us most. Our passion shines through on social media and flavors the digital content we gather, create, and share. Exploring the web for helpful sites or embarking on a writing project feels easy and fun when we are passionate about the topic.

Of course, our passions will only carry us so far, and often the topics we want to talk about are not the topics of interest to our patients and social media followers. So, after exhausting our go-to items, it's time to put our followers first and provide them with the answers they seek. Identifying these topics is easy. We simply pay attention to our followers' comments, questions, and shared content. How can we answer their questions and, more importantly, guide them toward greater understanding and an action plan? Think too about the questions clinic patients are asking. There are predictable patterns to these questions, and as folks begin asking their seasonal questions in person, you can bet our social media followers have the same questions in mind.

Where do we go when questions run dry? Fortunately, there are many places to discover ideas. Even though our followers are not discussing a particular topic, we can spark their interest and answer questions they had not considered. In many cases, this ignites new conversation, and our followers appreciate the awareness we create. One way to find an idea is to Google a specialty and click on the "news" tab in the results. What are mainstream news outlets currently covering? What articles appear from specialty publications? Can we present a topic aimed at our colleagues and spin the material for a different audience? As medical professionals, we have the knowledge and skills to evaluate and translate scientific articles in many disciplines and provide an understandable and practical commentary for our followers. Additional evidence-based resources can extend our knowledge as we strive to help others understand. These include PubMed, Google Scholar, UpToDate, DynaMed, and the Cochrane Collaboration.

Many professional organizations, such as the American Academy of Pediatrics and the American Medical Association, maintain a daily email digest with links to current topics of interest to consumers and medical professionals. If your area of interest has one of these, be sure to subscribe! Websites that aggregate current

Table 5.2 Ways to generate topic ideas

10 places to find topic ideas
1. Inside your mind – What are your interests and passions?
2. The examination room – What questions are your patients asking?
3. Your social media feeds – What are your followers talking about?
4. The mainstream news media – What headlines are circulating?
5. Peer-reviewed journals – What are your colleagues discussing?
6. PubMed.gov – What are hot topics of research in your specialty?
7. SmartBrief.com – Get a daily email digest of news in your field.
8. EurekAlert.org – Discover press releases for your area of interest.
9. MedicalNewsToday.com – Daily health and medical news.
10. HealthDay.com – Daily health and medical news.

medical news can also be helpful. Examples include Medical News Today, HealthDay, and Physician's Briefing. These are organized by specialty and feature articles based on recently published peer-reviewed research. Not only is this a terrific way to stay current in our field of practice, it also provides ideas for content that may be new and helpful for our followers. In addition to raising awareness about a particular article, this presents an opportunity to describe the strength of evidence, which might not be great. We can explain how the research fits in with what is already known, consider next steps for future research, and provide practical tips (if any) for using the new knowledge to improve health and wellness.

When choosing a topic based on current research, look for a press release from the originating academic institution or the journal itself. A great place to find these is the EurekAlert! website. Simply search for the name of the article or an author. This will give you a nice summary of the research project, along with quotes you can use if you are writing a blog post or creating other forms of digital content. Of course, best understanding of the work comes from reading the article's abstract and full text from the journal. This is the best way to truly grasp the research and its implications. Table 5.2 highlights various ways to develop topic ideas.

Why Do We Want Them to Know?

Understanding why we want to share a particular topic is as important as choosing it in the first place. In fact, after considering "why," we may elect to skip the topic and move on to something else. The first questions we should ask are will this topic be useful for improving health and wellness, what behaviors are we hoping to change, and what health outcomes are we looking to improve? Our topic should matter to someone. It should make a difference. Otherwise, we are contributing to the digital noise. It is fairly easy to spin most topics into usefulness. Even poorly designed research can be useful as we educate consumers and our colleagues about the paper's real implications and how that might differ from what mainstream media is reporting. Sometimes our call to action is that patients and families should take no action at all.

Next, it is important for us to examine the collective strength of evidence behind our thoughts, even when we think we are experts and know the answer. What do other experts think and why? What evidence has come before and what further evidence do we need to obtain? Healthcare consumers and our colleagues are placing trust in what we are sharing and saying, so it's important to get this right. Sometimes this search strengthens our resolve. Other times it raises questions about our own understanding. This is a good thing! How can we expect our followers to understand research findings and potentially change behaviors when we are not certain ourselves? When areas are gray, it is okay to say so. Our followers appreciate transparent honesty and are more likely to trust us on future topics when we speak the truth, even when the truth is "I don't know the answer."

Once we determine that our topic is useful and reflects current evidence, it is time to develop tangible goals surrounding it. Think specifically about how you want to raise awareness, change (or not change) behavior and alter health and wellness. For example, if our topic is asthma, what specific goals do we have? There are many to choose from, and while it's good to cover many of the reporter questions to provide framework and understanding, it's also important to identify specific goals within the broader topic. For example, we may want to raise awareness of the difference between daily controller medications and rescue inhalers, encourage our followers to use them correctly, and decrease the number and severity of asthma exacerbations because they put their knowledge into action. This line of thinking can become the focus of our effort, even as we explain risks, triggers, symptoms, and prevention as background information.

Who Do We Want to Tell?

After we select a topic and establish goals, it is time to determine who we want to tell. This group is our target audience. Identifying a specific target audience is important because the most effective way of telling a story may differ greatly from one audience to another. An obvious target audience may come immediately to mind, but it is important to think about less obvious choices too. We can sometimes make an unexpected impact by selecting a peripheral group. For example, as we think about asthma education, patients or parents of children with asthma immediately come to mind. However, there are many groups who can impact health outcomes when we empower them with knowledge related to asthma. Babysitters, daycare workers, and teachers need to know early signs of an asthma exacerbation, so they can administer or direct kids to use their rescue inhaler. Physical educations teachers, coaches, and athletic trainers benefit from information on exercise-induced asthma, and we can remind physicians, nurse practitioners, and medical learners the importance of early steroid administration when children present with significant symptoms.

With our target audience in mind, we can lay the foundation of our story's framework. This may result in altered goals depending on the audience we choose. That's okay! Without submitting ourselves to the process, we may easily overlook an important audience that could make a difference if we are willing to engage them. Identifying our target audience also helps us choose the words we use and how we use them. Will we employ plain language, technical terms, or a combination of the two? Toward what grade level will we write? Will we lean toward complex sentences or simple ones? How many words will we use? Will we break them into manageable segments (like this chapter) or create uninterrupted, lengthy prose? What tone will we take? Will we speak from a place of unwavering authority or express empathy for different positions? What sort of support can we offer and how can we best provide it?

Identifying the target audience also helps us determine the format of our content. Will we simply engage with brief comments, posts or tweets? Would a blog post work better? What about a podcast or colorful infographic? Shared news stories, Pinterest boards, magazine articles, press releases, technical reports, and journal articles are other possibilities. If we are sharing curated content, it is important to determine if the intended audience is similar to ours. For example, it is unlikely babysitters would benefit from a shared journal article, while out colleagues certainly would.

Finally, our target audience determines where we should engage. Where in the digital landscape do members of our audience hang out? Is there a Facebook page or Twitter account that caters to babysitters? What about blogs aimed at teachers? Perhaps we could write a guest post or offer an interview to the author, so she can write a post of her own. Can we find a sports medicine podcast with an audience full of coaches and athletic trainers? Podcast producers are always looking for unique content and opportunities to interview experts! Once the interview is recorded, we can share the episode with Facebook pages and Twitter account that cater to athletes, coaches, and trainers. If our target audience is colleagues or learners, where can we effectively engage them? Many possibilities exist, including the Facebook pages, Twitter accounts, blogs and podcasts of influential peers, journals, academic institutions, hospitals, and professional organizations.

Sometimes, we want to engage more than one target audience with a particular topic. While this is a fine idea, we must consider each audience on its own merits and carefully design unique engagement strategies. There are added benefits of identifying multiple target audiences and seeking them out. The process often leads us to digital landscapes we have not visited before, places outside our comfort zone. However, these are places that can lead to new perspectives. We may discover novel myths, complicated challenges, or unexpected barriers that force us to alter the course of our narrative as we strive to help and support our newfound friends. For instance, in helping teachers learn the early symptoms of an asthma exacerbation, we may discover school rules in certain locations prevent quick access to rescue medication. Thus, new target audiences are born: legislators and school officials who make the rules.

As our story unfolds with new audiences and strategies, the true nature of our work becomes clear. We are child advocates who are making a difference. We are shaping outcomes, gaining friends, increasing our following, and securing a reputation for providing trustworthy information.

How Can We Best Tell Them?

In addition to providing evidence-based trustworthy information, we must also strive to be practical and helpful. This means assessing the needs of our target audience and providing tips and tools that convert recommendations into action. The identified needs of our audience can relate to the outcome goal itself, or it may be something that grabs their attention and encourages them to engage. Either way, the needs assessment will play a major role in determining how we tell our story.

Let's consider parents of kids with asthma as our target audience. Our goal is help them understand the difference between controller and rescue medication and when to use each. What do parents need to achieve this goal? One idea is to put an asthma action plan into their hands. So, instead of just telling them when to use each, we are providing a tool that helps them do it. We don't have to create one of our own (although we could). There are plenty of easy-to-use asthma action plans available for immediate download, and we can provide a link as we comment, post, or tweet. If we do not like the idea of a paper plan, we can provide a link to an asthma mobile app that incorporates an action plan in the design.

What if our target audience is babysitters or daycare workers? An infographic demonstrating the early signs of an asthma attack and suggested interventions would be helpful. This is something daycare workers could easily print and post. If we are inclined to produce the infographic, great! If not, we could easily find and share the link of an existing one. Coaches and trainers would benefit from a tip sheet and practical action plan for exercise-induced asthma, which they can share with additional coaching staff, student athletes, and families. This not only reinforces staff knowledge of the condition, it empowers them to teach their own audience (students and families) and provide them with something useful.

Sharing a tip sheet on the proper use of a metered-dose inhaler (MDI) and the importance of attaching a spacer helps teachers in the classroom. When a student pulls out an MDI, the teacher can monitor technique and provide teaching when needed. If MDIs are prohibited in the classroom and locked away in the office, sharing state laws and school-district policies that permit children to carry rescue inhalers and use them in the classroom can be a catalyst for discussion and eventual policy change in other jurisdictions and districts.

What if our target audience is medical colleagues or learners? Curating or creating practice toolkits surrounding asthma can be quite helpful. Perhaps we can find a CME activity to share, one that looks at the evidence for providing oral steroids sooner rather than later during an acute exacerbation. Clinicians need CME. So, by sharing the link we are meeting a need that encourages our colleagues to dig deeper into the content.

Identifying audience need and linking it to our goals requires creativity and a few extra steps. However, this is an important part of the storytelling process and time well spent. The more effort we put into encouraging behavior change in easy and practical ways, the more likely it is that these changes will take root and eventually impact health outcomes.

It's Story Time!

Let's regroup and consider how the first four reporter questions can help us build a complete story. We begin with a tale about asthma, but rather than concentrating on all aspects of the disease, we decide to narrow our focus to the important difference between controller medications and rescue inhalers. Parents of children with asthma will be our target audience, and we can easily pull them in by describing the fate of little Sam. The boy had run out of his red inhaler last winter, but he was doing well with the blue one, so his parents did not get a refill. Since he did not need the red one anymore, they decided to try him without the blue one too, and he continued doing well. Yay! He no longer needed medicine for his asthma, but they kept the blue inhaler around just in case. Then viral season returned, and Sam started wheezing. No problem. The blue inhaler worked before, so they started using it again…. except it did not work this time, despite his parents giving it twice a day as instructed on the label. Then they recall he can actually use the inhaler every 4 hours when wheezing gets bad, and Sam's wheezing was definitely getting worse. They decided to use the blue inhaler every 4 hours overnight and take him to the hospital if he did not improve by morning. Unfortunately, Sam was not better in the morning. He was worse. So, off the family goes to the emergency room, where Sam was started on oxygen, given a series of breathing treatments with "a different medication" and admitted to the inpatient ward for continued treatment. Sam pulled through, but his parents were very worried about their little boy. Some kids are not as lucky as Sam. Many are admitted to the intensive care unit. A few even die.

What was the parents' mistake? They confused their son's "blue" steroid inhaler with his "red" albuterol one. This provides an opportunity to explain the difference between controller and rescue medications in asthma. In explaining how each works, we can elaborate on the mechanisms by which asthma symptoms develop. We can reinforce when each type of medication is needed and help parents anticipate when there could be a problem, even when no symptoms are apparent. Finally, we can introduce the asthma action plan as a tool for keeping the inhalers straight, knowing when to use each and who to call or where to go if symptoms do not improve or get worse. Including a link to an asthma action plan and instructing readers to ask their primary care provider to customize it are icing on the cake.

Our story draws the reader in with a fictional account that triggers an emotional response and makes the message matter. It answers the questions who, what, when, where, why, and how and presents a call to action in the form of a helpful tool that encourages parents to put their new knowledge into practice. We could easily present this as a 500-word blog or Facebook post divided into five sections of roughly 100-words each.

1. The story of little Sam, including his experience in the emergency department.
2. An introduction of asthma and how controller and rescue medications work.
3. Early and late signs of asthma exacerbation.
4. What to do, who to call, and where to go when asthma gets worse.
5. Description of the asthma action plan, including links to an electronic version. We conclude with a description of Sam's outcome, how it could have been worse, and the role of the action plan in preventing severe symptoms.

This is just one example from our brief brainstorming session. We might choose a different focus or target audience. We could expand the topic with a series of posts or use a different story format, including podcasts, videos, infographics, or a series of short tweets. Another option is to curate content from other sources and strategically share these resources to tell our story.

When Is the Best Time to Tell Our Story?

The medical stories we create and share are often seasonal, so we must pay attention to yearly shifts in illness, injury, and wellness to remain relevant and beneficial. For example, swimming safety and nutritious outdoor grilling make sense in summer, while influenza and healthy chili recipes garner more interest in fall and winter. Seasonal allergies are big in the spring, hand-foot-mouth disease spikes in summer, croup is common in fall, and frostbite concerns mount as the weather turn cold. Despite these general observations, we must also keep our audience in mind. If we have an international crowd, seasons are flipped for some of our followers, and water safety works in the winter if we spin our coverage toward those participating in swim clubs and indoor aquatic facilities.

We can also take advantage of the many health awareness months. A sampling of these include Heart Month and Cancer Prevention Month in February, Kidney Month in March, Stress Awareness and Autism Awareness in April, Healthy Vision Month in May, Men's Health Month in June, Immunization Awareness Month in August, Breast Cancer Awareness in October, and Diabetes Month in November. Some awareness activities only last a week or on a specific day. For example, Hand Washing Awareness Week occurs in early December and World Mental Health Day is October 10th. Focusing on a single aspect of an awareness month and tailoring it for a specific target audience are great ways to serve the digital community.

It also helps to pay attention to news reports at the community, state, national, and international levels. When we read or hear stories about an infectious disease outbreak, natural disaster, or terror attack, we can use the opportunity to consider how the event impacts health and wellness and how we can support our followers with reassurance and advice rooted in evidence and experience. This is a good time to mention that being an expert on a particular topic is not required for us to chime in on social media. In addition to being experts in specific disciplines, we are also experts at finding and interpreting the best information available. For instance, the Centers for Disease Control and Prevention will have terrific information on the diagnosis and management of an emerging disease, the Federal Emergency Management Agency will have tips for those who have experienced a hurricane, and the Department of Homeland Security will share important information following a terror attack. Our experience in fact-checking and hunting down the best evidence and information as we gather, share, and interpret on a regular basis prepares us to become content experts on any topic when unexpected tragedy strikes. We are enabled and should be ready to engage with relevant and beneficial content at a moment's notice, even when the topic is not part of our everyday medical practice.

In addition to the news cycle, we should continuously monitor our social media feeds, paying attention to the questions our followers are asking and the content they are sharing. Any topic is timely when it attracts attention, whatever the reason. Those with questions will find answers somewhere. It is better that answers come from us, even if we were not planning on covering a particular topic at a particular time. While we may strive to create editorial calendars for our content, ultimately those we serve have an important say in what we say and when we say it.

Finally, it's okay to repeat content we have already shared, especially when the story becomes relevant and beneficial again. Last year's blog post on Lyme disease is fine to reshare on Facebook or Twitter when the disease returns for another season. Likewise, an article about a parent's response to her child's questions following a school shooting is helpful each and every time a school shooting occurs.

Where Is the Best Place to Tell Our Story?

The first place we typically tell our story is within our everyday digital habitat. We share it with our followers on social media. If we have a blog or podcast or YouTube channel, we share it there. In many cases, this is enough. Our target audience lives among our followers, and we succeed in raising awareness, promoting health and wellness, and reaching our goals through this ordinary means. However, at other times, we can serve a greater good when we move out of our comfort zone and seek the target audience in new locations.

So, how do we find a target audience? One way is to put ourselves in their shoes and try to think like they would think. Where do they hang out? What questions are they asking? Search for online sites or digital media that cater to our target audience, and spend some time reading and watching. As we get comfortable with the culture, we can begin engaging. We can make note of the questions our target audience is asking. Search Google for the answers and see what sort of information is out there. Is it good and helpful information or full of myths and misconceptions? As we engage, try to identify specific needs of the target audience. The more time we spend getting to know them, the easier it will be to identify a need. Then we can search for a resource that will help. If we cannot find an adequate resource, it may be time to create something new!

Finally, we share our story with the target audience and connect them with our helpful resources. In this way, we are doing far more than stating facts and offering unsolicited advice. We are a member of the group. We have their best interest in mind. We are ready to raise awareness and truly help. Of course, this sort of engagement takes time. We may be cultivating several different audiences with unique topics and goals on any given day. It may take a few days or even weeks before we are ready to engage and share. But the results are worth the wait, especially when we are able to provide something useful to those in need, something that will change their trajectory of health and wellness.

What does this look like from a practical standpoint? Let's choose a new target audience for our campaign to raise awareness on the proper use of rescue inhalers in asthma. How about school teachers? We begin by thinking like a teacher. Where might teachers hang out? A Google search takes us to a Reddit board for teachers with over 80,000 subscribers, including over 500 online at the current time. Being a teacher is not a requirement to join, so we do. We read through some of the posts, to get a sense of community, and discover a post from a teacher who asks other teachers if they carry an asthma inhaler with them in the classroom. We chime in with a question, "Just curious. Are students allowed to carry rescue inhalers in your school?" This sparks a conversation! One teacher reports students can, while another says students must go to the office where the inhaler is locked away. A third teacher grumbles about school administration not understanding the importance of quick treatment with a rescue inhaler. Another teacher voices fear that she cannot tell if students are using the inhaler properly. She prefers students have nurse supervision. Finally, a teacher wishes there were written guidelines all schools could follow.

A quick Google search reveals a document from the American Lung Association called "Improving Access to Asthma Medications in Schools." It presents evidence supporting self-carry by students and outlines a plan schools can adopt to do this safely, including permission from parents, permission from the child's doctor, an asthma action plan on file with the school, and the student's ability to demonstrate proper use of the inhaler. The document also considers liability protection for the school and its staff. We share the document with the group, mention being a medical provider, and offer a quick story about a recent patient who ended up on 5 days of steroids following a delay in using his inhaler at school. We end by inviting questions regarding rescue inhalers and asthma action plans.

This example took no more than an hour of our time and offered helpful evidence-based advice in a location visited by thousands of members of our target audience. Perhaps we will have future opportunities to engage teachers in this newfound forum.

Engage the Audience

Telling a story through simple engagement is a powerful means of communication. There is no need to tell our entire story at once. Through posts and tweets and comments and shares, we can reveal the many components of our story over time. The result is a tale that builds upon itself. We can lay a foundation, introduce concepts, construct a frame, fill it with facts, and empower our audience with tools and resources. This can occur in a natural and organic way over a short or long period of time. Details emerge as we cultivate relationships and build trust. These are important jobs because our audience will certainly come across information that conflicts with ours, but it is our content we want them to grasp and remember and act upon.

Although stories presented through social media engagement tend to be fragmented, it remains important to plan the entire story at the front end. This helps us avoid stale repetition. New posts can introduce fresh perspective as we consider each of the reporter questions in turn. The end result provides our audience with greater understanding and a clear call to action.

In addition to storytelling, we can expand our knowledge through social media engagement, which is an important part of the professional life. Exposure to ideas that challenge our opinion is a good thing. It forces us to consider why we believe and recommend as we do. Challenge encourages us to check our facts and explain things in a different way. Fact-checking reinforces our understanding of the science, and figuring out new ways to explain something makes future engagement more efficient and effective. Both of these actions benefit our future followers and our clinic patients. Challenge should result in a change in our opinions and advice if we uncover fresh facts rooted in strong peer-reviewed evidence. This is how we evolve as practitioners!

Finally, social media engagement gives us ideas for future stories. As we communicate with others, we will frequently feel passion rising about a particular topic of discussion. Our gut may tell us to jump right in, but a bit of research and planning before joining the conversation can strengthen the impact of our eventual involvement. It is also a good idea to curate content as we engage. What are others sharing right now that we could share in the future? Consider keeping a folder of digital resources that will stimulate and strengthen future stories.

Curate Great Content

Telling a story with curated content can be a fun and challenging exercise. The good news is that someone likely has thoughts and recommendations similar to our own. They may have created a fantastic piece of digital content to support their ideas, but the content has not gotten as much traction as they would like. We can help! Whether it is a blog post, news article, infographic, podcast episode, online video, webinar, or education module, content creators love when we share their stuff. Just be sure to provide links to the original material and give credit where credit is due. Likewise, we should consider it an honor when others share our work. We reach and impact the greatest number of people when we all work together and share each other's digital stuff.

As we curate and share the work of others, we must still pay attention to the story we want to tell. What goals do we have? Are these adequately addressed in the content? Why do we have these goals? What behavior or outcome do we wish to change? Who is the target audience? How can we meet their needs? When and where can we best engage? Unless the creator has paid attention to telling the same story we want to tell, it's unlikely that a single artifact will serve our purpose. Surely, we have more to say! Our well-developed story may include several pieces of curated content; a few tweets, posts, or comments; and, perhaps, a digital piece we create on our own.

See Chap. 7 for more details on content curation.

Create Great Content

Creating digital content takes time, effort, and skill. However, this form of engagement in the digital realm can also be greatly rewarding and impactful. Each form of created content presents a unique set of challenges. There are rules and conventions to learn. Technical considerations may be substantial, and in some cases, there is cost associated with hosting and distribution. Whether you are thinking about writing a blog post, recording a podcast, designing an infographic, or producing a video, the first order of business is to consume as many examples as we can. How have others managed the creation? What aspects do we like? What would we do differently? We can also seek out instruction. There are plenty of blogs that teach blog writing, podcasts that teach podcasting, infographics that explain how to put one together, and video tutorials on creating videos. Take advantage of the insider tips these resources provide.

If you are not ready to create your own content, but still have a need for something new, consider offering yourself as a content expert for someone else's work. You don't need your own blog to write a guest post or feed the blogger expert content for a particular post. Podcast producers are always looking for expert guests, and podcasts can offer some very specific target audiences. For example, we could look for a podcast that targets school teachers. We simply pitch the idea of appearing as a guest. We can talk about asthma inhalers, outline the importance of self-carry for rescue inhalers and discuss guidelines from the American Lung Association on implementing school policy. In addition to reaching the podcast audience, we can amplify the message with our own followers (and among teachers on our new-found Reddit board) by simply sharing the link to the episode. Offering ourselves to local television and radio stations can also work as many broadcast outlets share their on-air content as podcasts and videos, furthering the reach and impact our message can have.

A local artist (maybe your son or daughter) could create a compelling infographic. Speaking of our kids and teens, they might know a lot more about video production than we do. Perhaps they could teach us how to record and set up a YouTube channel. From there, we can easily share our educational videos on Facebook, Twitter, and other social media sites.

Like our curated content, it remains important to think about the story we want to tell as we create. Will our piece encapsulate the entire story or serve a small part of something bigger? There are no right or wrong answers to this question, and herein lies the joy of online engagement and digital content production. We are making the rules as we go. We are the pioneers and trail-blazers. It is okay to experiment and have fun in the process! See Fig. 5.1 for medically specific examples of

Medical storytelling

	HPV vaccine	Flu shot	Gluten-free	Fluoride
Anecdote-based stories				
Hook	HPV vaccine causes brain damage	Flu shot results in illness and hurts immunity	Gluten causes brain fog and ADHD	Fluoride causes cancer
Why it matters	Here's what happened to my child	Here's my experience	Here's our before and after story	Look what happened to these people
Call to action	Skip this vaccine!	Don't get a flu shot!	Go gluten-free!	Vote "no" on adding fluoride to city water!
Evidence-based stories				
Hook	HPV causes deadly cancers	It's that time of year	Sleep helps brain fog and ADHD	Pictures of severe tooth decay and gingivitis
Why it matters	HPV vaccine safely prevents many cancers	185 children died from flu last season	Brain fog and ADHD affect quality of life	There is an easy way to prevent tooth deccay
Call to action	Get an HPV vaccine!	Get a flu shot!	Get more sleep!	Vote "yes" on the levy!

Planning a medical story

	HPV vaccine	Flu shot	Gluten-free	Fluoride
WHAT Message	HPV vaccine is safe and prevents cancer	Flu shots are not 100% effective, but they do save lives	Gluten is unlikely to cause ADHD or behavior problems	Fluoride in water is safe and prevents tooth decay
Why Goals	Increase HPV vaccine uptake and prevent cancer	Increase flu shot uptake and prevent flu deaths	Maintain healthy nutrition and use startegies that work	Prevent morbidity associated with dental carries
Who Target audience	Parents of pre-teens	Everyone	Parents of kids with ADHD	Voters
How Meet needs	Share vaccine schedule and outline benefits for girls and boys	Explain post-shot symptoms and need for yearly injection	Share sleep hygiene tips and explain how ADHD medicines work	Explain how fluoride works and provide safe exposure levels
When Message timing	Any time of the year	Early fall	During the school year	Before the vote
Where Digital activity	Blog post YouTube video Curate / share content	Infographic Blog post Podcast interview	Engage followers YouTube video Blog post	Local newspaper op-ed Local radio interview Infographic

Fig. 5.1 Examples of how to use storytelling related to health information

how to employ storytelling in dissemination of evidence-based information. Chapter 8 has an in-depth discussion of ways to curate new content.

Putting It All together

Let's complete our journey in the art of digital storytelling with one more exercise.

In the course of looking for a topic to share, I consult one of my go-to medical news aggregators, a website called Medical News Today. In the pediatrics section, I discover a story about regular fish consumption being associated with increased sleep quality and higher IQ [1]. Before sharing this story with my audience, I want to know more about the researchers and the science. I search for the authors and the topic on EurekAlert! and read the press release about the project [2]. Satisfied by that report, I search for the article itself in the journal *Scientific Reports*.

The article, "Effects of Weekly Fish Consumption on IQ and Sleep Quality," [3] was published in December 2017 and comes from the University of Pennsylvania. I am satisfied by the strength of evidence, which reveals that weekly fish intake is associated with a statistically significant improvement in sleep and IQ scores. Additionally, the improved quality of sleep further enhances the improved IQ. The authors recommend parents encourage children to eat more fish based on the results of their work. This recommendation seems like a good idea to me, especially since other studies have demonstrated additional health benefits of increasing fish consumption compared to other meats.

So, thinking about the reporter questions, what do I want people to know and why do I want them to know? Pretty easy. I want children and teens to eat more fish because that might improve their sleep, IQ, and other health determinants. Okay, who do I want to tell? There are many good choices for my target audience. I may want parents to know. Medical colleagues and learners should know, so they can educate patients and followers about the findings. Those in charge of designing school lunches ought to know. After all, if parents are not feeding kids fish at home, perhaps schools will do it.

After careful consideration, I decide to make parents my target audience. However, in an effort to focus on a more specific audience, I choose parents with toddlers. This seems like a good idea because if moms and dads can get toddlers to eat fish regularly, perhaps it will propel these children toward regular fish-eating the rest of their lives. Plus, by choosing a very specific target audience, I can narrow down their needs and consider how I might best help them.

So, what do parents of toddlers need as they think about increasing fish consumption at family meals? After a brief brainstorming session, I come up with three ideas.

1. Young kids may resist the taste of fish, so parents may need ideas on tasty kid-friendly recipes.
2. Fish can be expensive compared to other options, so parents may need ideas for buying fish on a budget.
3. Parents might be concerned about toxins, such as mercury, in fish. They may like reassurance and guidance on eating fish safely.

With these ideas in mind, I could easily create a short blog post with an introduction, three major sections, a conclusion, and a few links to curated content that helps parents overcome the barriers of taste, cost, and toxins. But before I do that, let me consider when and where I want to tell my story. The topic is not seasonal, so now is a good time. Where? Instead of immediately writing a blog post, I could begin at home, in my social media channel. I could engage my followers with a link to the original news story, followed by comments summarizing the science. I could encourage parents of toddlers to offer their kids more fish, outline the barriers, and provide links to resources that help parents overcome each one. I could accomplish this as a series of short posts, comments, or tweets over the course of several hours or days.

I could also look for digital communities with large numbers of my target audience. I do a Google search for "encourage kids to eat fish" and one of the first results is an article in Parenting magazine called "6 Ways to Encourage Your Child to Eat Fish." [4] Okay, I wonder if Parenting magazine is on Twitter. Yes, it is! In fact, they have over two million followers [5], many of whom are parents of toddlers who would be interested in my message! I write a tweet that states the associations between eating fish, sleeping, and IQ. I include a link to the news story and call out Parenting magazine by including their handle (@parenting) in my tweet. I also call out @ModernMom (412,000 followers) [6] and @PlaygroundDad (347,000 followers) [7] because the Parenting magazine Twitter page told me these are accounts I might also like. Finally, I add a hashtag (#EatMoreFish) that promises to gain more attention.

Out goes my tweet. It gets some likes and retweets, and I gain a few more followers. If @Parenting, @ModernMom or @PlaygroundDad decide to like or retweet my message, I'll get more traction. As it turns out, they do not engage me, but a couple Twitter users comment on my post. One mentions how difficult it is to get her toddler to eat fish. I share a link from Martha Stewart: "Kid-Friendly Fish and Shell-Fish Recipes" [8] and another from MyFussyeater.com: "10 Kid-Approved Fish Recipes." [9] More users like and retweet my reply. Others comment with their own kid-friendly fish recipes. Before I know it, there is an entire conversation taking place below my tweet! I respond to all the commenters with another tweet stating fish is expensive. This gets several likes. Another user shares a link to a blog post called "Buying Healthy Fish on a Budget." [10] I had not seen that one, but I look it up and the post has some great advice. I save the link, so I can include it as a resource in my eventual blog post.

I am about to give up on the conversation when another user chimes in, "Is fish safe for kids to eat?" I jump at the opportunity and find and share a link from Parents Magazine called "Which Fish are Safe for Kids?" [11] and another from HealthyChildren.org called "Healthy Fish Choices for Kids," which includes information on protecting children from contaminated fish [12]. The user thanks me and I call it a night on Twitter. In the meantime, various pieces of the conversation have been retweeted and commented on by others. Some add more links to helpful sites. Retweets are retweeted by others. By morning, I check the impressions and see my original tweet has been seen by nearly 2000 people. Many of them will have followed the entire conversation. This is pretty good reach for 30 minutes of my time. I do not know if anyone will give their kids more fish based on my effort, but it sure is a nice start for raising awareness.

A few days later, I write my blog post and share it with my followers on Facebook and Twitter. The article begins with a hook, and I strive to make the message matter before presenting my call to action. The post gets many likes and shares. A few readers thank me. As a result of my blog post, parents of toddlers have heard an important message. I have anticipated their needs and shared a wealth of resources that provide tasty fish recipes on a budget and with safety in mind. Compare this effort to simply tweeting the original news article with a brief comment that says, "eat more fish" and then moving on to something else. Which strategy is more likely to change behavior and improve outcomes? The scientific literature does not have an answer to this question, but experience and intuition tell me creating a story is more impactful and worth the effort.

Conclusion

We are most engaged with content when information is presented as a story. Medical myths and misconceptions are often perpetuated by those who use storytelling elements to relate anecdotal information and experiences. They hook their audience, trigger an emotional response, and present what appears to be a quite reasonable call to action. If medical professionals are to effectively counter these inaccurate messages, we too must become passionate storytellers. We must draw people in and establish a connection. We must let folks know we care as we share and explain the evidence. We must strive to be relevant and beneficial and useful. In this way, we can harness the power of storytelling to make a very real difference in the lives of many.

References

1. Whiteman H. Eating fish weekly improves kids' sleep, intelligence. Medical News Today, December 2017. https://www.medicalnewstoday.com/articles/320441.php.
2. Weekly fish consumption linked to better sleep, higher IQ, Penn study finds. EurekAlert!, December 2017. https://www.eurekalert.org/pub_releases/2017-12/uop-wfc121917.php.
3. Liu J, et al. The mediating role of sleep in the fish consumption – cognitive functioning relationship: a cohort study. Scientific reports, December 2017. https://www.nature.com/articles/s41598-017-17520-w.
4. Rhodes M. 6 ways to encourage your child to eat fish. Parenting. 2018. https://www.parenting.com/article/6-ways-to-encourage-your-child-to-eat-fish.
5. @Parenting. Twitter. 2018. https://twitter.com/parenting?lang=en.
6. @Modernmom. Twitter. 2018. https://twitter.com/ModernMom?lang=en.
7. @Playgrounddad. Twitter. 2018. https://twitter.com/playgrounddad?lang=en.
8. Kid-friendly fish and shellfish recipes. Martha Stewart. 2018. https://www.marthastewart.com/339169/kid-friendly-fish-and-shellfish-recipes.
9. Attwell C. 10 kid-approved fish recipes. My fussy eater, June 2018. https://www.myfussyeater.com/10-kid-approved-fish-recipes/.
10. Buying healthy fish on a budget. Sara Snow. 2018. https://sarasnow.com/buying-healthy-fish-on-a-budget/.
11. Kuzemchak S. Which fish are safe for kids? Parents, June 2015. https://www.parents.com/blogs/food-scoop/2015/06/30/nutrition/which-fish-are-safe-for-kids/.
12. Healthy fish choices for kids. HealthyChildren. 2018. https://www.healthychildren.org/English/safety-prevention/all-around/Pages/Protecting-Your-Children-From-Contaminated-Fish.aspx.

If You Tweet It, They Will Come

6

David R. Stukus

> *LinkedIn is for the people you know. Facebook is for the people you used to know. Twitter is for people you want to know*

> —Source unknown

Start with Your Profile

The home page in Twitter is where your followers or anyone who lands on your handle will first learn about you. With limited attention spans and lots of competition, the first impression you make on others is extremely important. The handle on Twitter refers to the name of your account. All Twitter handles are preceded by the "@" symbol and then can include any string of characters the user wishes to use. Healthcare professionals must decide whether they are using Twitter for professional or personal purposes, or both. It helps to search other accounts with similar interests to see what grabs your attention and also what is already taken. Users can change their handle anytime and not lose followers; everything on their account will remain linked, which removes some of the pressure of needing to choose the *perfect* handle at the outset. When choosing your handle, consider how you want to represent yourself to the rest of the Twitter world. You can include your name, or some variation thereof, or your area of interest. Using random wording or a long sequence of numbers is not advised as this will not communicate who you are or why you are present on social media.

There are many examples of healthcare-related Twitter accounts that have a large number of followers and a wide-ranging influence. Some use their own names, while others use humor or more applicable topics of interest. When deciding upon a handle, consider what is available, what message you want to convey, and what makes the most sense for your personality. When I first joined Twitter in 2013, I had a desire to use social media to disseminate evidence-based medicine surrounding asthma, a condition that I was focused on clinically and with my

© Springer Nature Switzerland AG 2019
D. R. Stukus et al., *Social Media for Medical Professionals*,
https://doi.org/10.1007/978-3-030-14439-5_6

Table 6.1 Medical Twitter accounts with large number of followers

Account handle	Topics of interest	Number of followers[a]
@EricTopol	Medical informatics, technology	146,000
@DrJenGunter	Women's health, gynecology	103,000
@Atul_Gwande	Healthcare delivery	268,000
@medicalaxioms	Medical wisdom	51,300
@kevinmd	Various topics	156,000
@gruntdoc	Emergency medicine	12,200
@Doctor_V	Technology, social media	32,100

[a]As of December, 2018

research. Then, a conversation with a colleague changed my career forever. She suggested that I not limit myself to one topic, but to use social media to discuss all allergic and immunologic conditions. Thus, I went from my initial idea of becoming @AsthmaKidsDoc to @AllergyKidsDoc. This seemingly small change made an enormous difference. As @AllergyKidsDoc, I interact with the robust online food allergy community, who have a tremendous presence on Twitter, in particular. I also discuss drug allergy, venom allergy, hay fever, anaphylaxis, antibiotic stewardship, smoking cessation, etc. I also realized that by using "Allergy" at the front of my handle, I would show up in searches and place myself at the forefront of anyone looking for allergy-related information on Twitter. My personal example highlights how impactful the choice of a handle can be on establishing an audience. Table 6.1 lists several examples of successful medical Twitter accounts and demonstrates the range of handles that can be used.

The Twitter home page allows two photos to be used, which can be anything the user chooses. The circular profile picture is typically where people include a picture of themselves, which allows anyone who lands on their page to see who they are and what they look like. The background photograph runs across the top of the home page. This is an area where users can display their interests or display some creativity. The default profile picture for new Twitter users is an anonymous silhouette. All healthcare professionals who use Twitter should absolutely change the default profile picture! Nothing says "novice" like leaving the default in place. Most healthcare professionals use a professional portrait taken by their employer or another high-resolution personal photograph, but this is not mandatory for success (Fig. 6.1). Some medical Twitter accounts prefer to remain anonymous, particularly among medical students who fear their social media accounts may be subject to scrutiny as they move forward in their career. Of course, if professionalism standards are maintained, then no medical professionals should fear retribution for their social media posts.

Twitter allows a very useful tool for individual accounts through the profile feature on the home page. The profile is the character limited area where each account can relay whatever information they choose to help others learn about them very quickly. Healthcare professionals should think of this as their very brief "elevator speech" to tell the world who they are, why they are here, and what their interests are. Links to other Twitter accounts and use of hashtags can help increase visibility as well. This is the area where professional affiliations, location, interests, and creative wordsmithing can have an impact. Figure 6.2

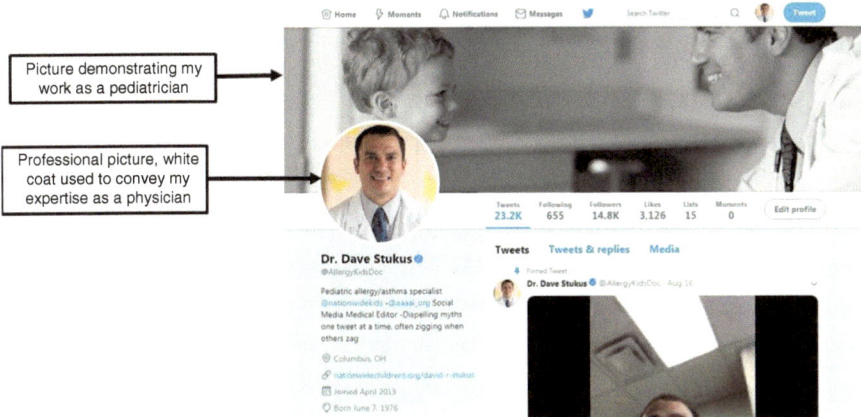

Fig. 6.1 Professional background and profile picture

Fig. 6.2 Twitter profiles highlight interests, professional affiliations and provide links to other sites

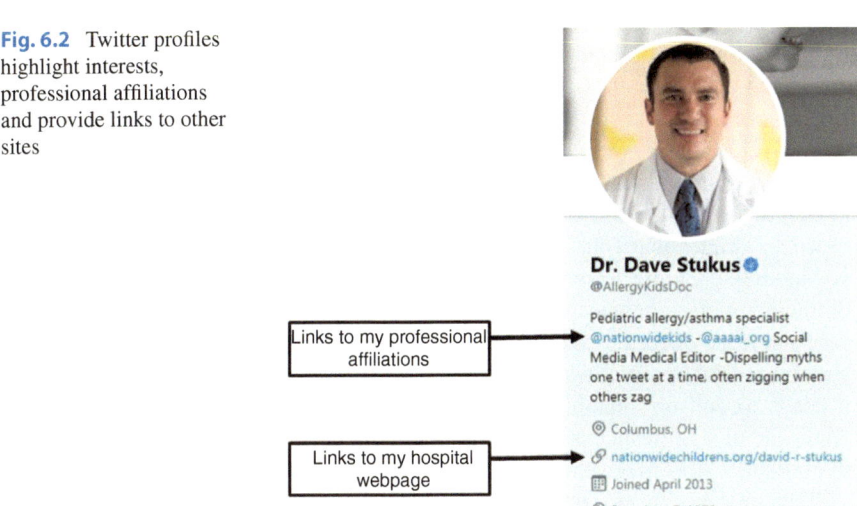

highlights my Twitter profile. As you see, I very clearly state my profession in the first line. I also include my hospital affiliation and role with my specialty's professional organization. This conveys that I am an academician and involved on a national level with my professional organizations. One of my main interests in using social media is to provide evidence-based information but also combat misinformation, thus my tag line "Dispelling myths one tweet at a time." You can include links to other social media accounts or websites within the Twitter profile, as I have done to direct people to my hospital webpage where they can see my publications, education, and background.

It is worth the time and thoughtfulness to develop a professional-appearing home page. Whether first starting out on Twitter, or editing a current home page, consider what message you want to send to new followers or those who land on your account through searching for information or being directed when someone else retweets your posts. View this as a prime opportunity to introduce yourself to a new user and grab their attention. Is your account colorful, vibrant, and professional-appearing? This conveys the sense that you are not only a professional but that you are dedicated to providing quality information. Or is your home page not current, dull, or bare? This conveys that you are absent for long stretches and not dedicated to providing quality information or discussion.

Consider Your Audience Before Yourself

Bryan Vartabedian is a gastroenterologist in Texas who has developed a multifaceted social media presence. In addition to his Twitter account @Doctor_V, he has a website 33charts.com that is used to post his own blogs as well as assemble articles from across medicine [1]. His Twitter profile states that his account "Dispatches from the frontline of technology and medicine" and his target audience is mainly healthcare professionals, but information is posted in a manner that patients and the general public may relate to as well. One of his blog posts centered on building a target audience and offers wonderful insight for medical professionals (or anyone) who are building their social media platform [2]. In lieu of focusing on getting the most retweets, followers, or likes, you should instead focus on providing something of *value*. Think about your own habits and interests when spending time online. Are you more likely going to spend time reading an article or website, follow an account, or interact with someone else if they are providing valuable content that aligns with your interests, or if they are merely providing more noise in a world already filled with noise? As Dr. Vartabedian writes "When you commit to writing or recording, it needs to deliver something that helps your reader or viewer. *It's about value.* Audience of significance is earned and should never be assumed. And it takes years of consistent stuff to develop even a small following."

Take time to consider who your target audience is going to be and how you can best connect with them. It is perfectly fine to have multiple different target audiences, and for your audience to change over time. It is also helpful to consider that not every post, article, blog, retweet, or comment will resonate with everyone. Trying to please all the people all the time will lead to diluted, less meaningful content. My audience for @AllergyKidsDoc on Twitter consists of patients, the general public, media, medical students, primary care clinicians, dietitians, allergists, and fellow myth busters. As you can imagine, that represents a wide range of backgrounds and interests. Some of my posts and content seem to resonate with all of these groups, whereas others are tailored to a very specific portion of my audience. I do try to consciously share content that each segment may find useful from time to time, in an effort to maintain relevance and provide value to all of my followers. However, I also do not force specific content just to check a box.

As you develop your social media presence and voice, consider the areas that you are passionate about and then seek like-minded individuals online. Through Twitter, you can search for similar topics, handles, or accounts that are posting similar information. You can then see who their followers are and the information they are posting as well. Connecting with these groups can be as simple as following these accounts, and they may reciprocate when they see the notification that you followed them. Similarly, if you retweet, like, or comment on their posts, they will also notice your account and may then follow you or reciprocate. Twitter is an amazing avenue for interaction and you can also ask accounts/individuals questions, reply to their questions/comments, or simply reach out to introduce yourself. The success of these strategies will vary by approach, timing, and the desire of the person on the receiving end to reciprocate, but by casting a wide net, you may establish meaningful connections.

Once you've got their attention…now what? This is where we need to circle back to providing value for your audience. If you spend time reaching out and establishing contacts on Twitter, then draw attention to your account…what will people find when they land there? Will they see a handle with meaningless numbers/characters, an empty silhouette in the profile picture, and limited content? Or will they discover a like-minded medical professional who has taken the time to cultivate a professional-appearing profile that describes who they are and why they're here, along with sharing of content that is useful and informative?

One of the great things about social media is the ability to reinvent oneself and grow over time. It is rare for someone to develop a social media account and gain one million followers instantly (Barack Obama came close). It is okay to change your pictures, your profile, and even your audience over time. There's a learning curve involved, which is part of the intellectual journey when using social media as a medical professional. But at every step along the way, try to remember the 5-second rule:

- If people don't find what they are looking for quickly, they will move on.
- Make a good first impression.
- Keep it short and simple (Twitter character limits are great at editing our long-winded thoughts).
- Keep it current and/or local (local can refer to geographic or within one's target audience).

One area many medical professionals struggle with when developing their social media presence is knowing what kind of information to post. Chapters 7 and 8 offer an in-depth discussion regarding content curation and creation. Twitter makes this easy, in some regards. The list of trending topics and hashtags is constantly refreshed. If something is trending that is related to your interests or target audience, that offers a great opportunity to post content, opinions, or share a blog post and insert yourself into the trending discussion which introduces your account to thousands of others looking at the same trending information at that time. You will see that the majority of those other accounts joining the trending conversation may have no interest in following a medical professional on Twitter, but even a few new followers will be worth the minimal effort it takes to capitalize on this unique Twitter feature. Other sources of inspiration for Twitter posts can include:

- Media reports – If you read an interesting article pertaining to your interests, share it with your followers. Better yet, provide your own comments regarding the applicability or limitations. This is particularly useful when media reports mischaracterize scientific studies or publications. As a medical professional, this is your area of expertise, and your followers will appreciate your insight.
- Journal articles – Many journals offer open access to their articles, which can be shared with your followers. This is how many medical professionals actually receive their own information, by following the Twitter account of medical journals or individuals who post high impact articles. Even if the entire article cannot be shared, you can provide a link to the PubMed page, which will have the abstract available for others to view. Again, providing commentary regarding study methodology, findings, and applicability can be a valuable addition to these posts.
- Personal experiences – As the medical professional, you are the expert. You can offer insight into the common clinical presentation, testing, and treatment of various conditions. Use your own patient care experiences to offer general medical information and even lessons learned from the front lines.
- Medical conferences – This is a growing area where Twitter is unparalleled. Most medical conferences will have a common hashtag that attendees can use to post information from sessions. This allows attendees to easily grow their social media presence among their colleagues, establish new connections, and network. It also provides information and opinions from thought leaders within a field for others to learn from, which is particularly valuable for anyone with interest but unable to attend the meeting. Larger meetings often see their conference hashtag trending during periods of high-volume tweeting, typically on the weekends.
- Conversations with friends, colleagues, and patients – If you have interesting discussion, questions, or clinical dilemmas, then take that information and turn it into a Twitter post, or series of posts. You can even pose it as a question or create a Twitter poll and ask people to provide their own answers. This can be a great way to increase engagement and establish yourself as a medical professional who is interested in online dialogue.
- Questions from real-life clinical encounters – If someone asks you a question, it is guaranteed that someone on social media has similar questions. Consider common areas of anticipatory guidance as well, even if these seem routine to your own practice. Remember, people are going online searching for medical information. If you are providing evidence-based information that pertains to their own condition and answers their questions, your followers will grow. It is useful to consider the various time points for those newly diagnosed, those with chronic conditions, acute exacerbations, and those who may have been cured.

This is another opportune time to reiterate the absolute necessity to maintain patient privacy at all times. I use personal encounters with patients for inspiration on a routine basis but try to never violate patient privacy. For example:

- A patient with peanut allergy asks if it is safe for them to eat tree nuts.
- Incorrect example to post: "A 16-year-old patient, who had anaphylaxis after eating peanut when he was 5, asked me today if he could eat tree nuts."
- Correct examples: "Peanuts are legumes. They do not naturally cross react with tree nuts. Tree nut allergies often occur in people with peanut allergy, but not due to cross reactivity" or "People with peanut allergy often avoid tree nuts as this is the safest way to avoid misidentification or cross contamination. However, many can safely find ways to eat tree nuts without problems."
- In each example, I would also provide a link to a blog post or article from a professional organization that offers a longer discussion surrounding this topic.

I first joined Twitter in 2013 and have spent years learning, changing, and adapting my approach. Many of my attempts have failed and did not resonate with my target audience, whereas others caught on and helped grow my following. With all of my effort and dedication, I have always tried to provide value for those who find my account and I have received wonderful feedback over the years about how the information I provide is either new, discussed in a way not previously understood, and generally helpful. I initially started and now continue with social media with the purpose of trying to help one patient, colleague, or person at a time, and the number of followers has never been a motivating factor. However, it is helpful to understand how this can grow one's platform and reach even more individuals. To offer some perspective, it took me nearly 5 years of providing content and conversation of value to reach 10,000 followers on Twitter. Again, not that this is a primary motivating factor, but this highlights the dedication and attention to providing value that is necessary to reach a wide audience. There are certainly many other medical professionals who have other areas of interest, wonderful personalities, or a strong media presence that have grown their audience much faster. But with time, dedication, and practice, anyone can build an audience…as long as you consider their needs before your own.

Think Like a Patient

One of the reasons I joined social media and Twitter in particular was due to the vast amounts of misinformation I was hearing from patients, colleagues, and media. I felt as though I had a firm grasp of the evidence surrounding many pediatric- and allergy-related conditions. Yet, the day-to-day management by referring clinicians and decisions made by patients often ignored or contradicted established evidence and clinical guidelines. It has been demonstrated that it takes up to 17 years for clinical guidelines to be implemented into practice [3]. There are multiple complicated and interconnected reasons for this, including inability of medical professionals to stay up to date with current research and guidelines, time constraints in a busy clinical setting, demands on time from the implementation of electronic medical records, lack of incentive, and continued belief in outdated teaching or practice styles. Those are just several reasons why medical professionals have a hard time staying up to date with their practice of medicine. Now we have social media and the Internet influencing our patient's beliefs, understanding, and decision-making. How do we stand a chance?

Medical professionals are generally trained in some regard about the scientific method, research methodology, and interpretation of statistics. Medical professionals learn early in their training that it is impossible for any one person to memorize, understand, and properly interpret ALL of the information necessary to practicing medicine. Thus, they learn how to search for and retrieve necessary information, often when the patient is present in the office or on bedside rounds. Medical professionals are trained in using vetted, evidence-based sources of information such as textbooks, Lexicomp for prescribing medications, UptoDate, or PubMed for searching peer-reviewed journals. When looking for the proper dose of amoxicillin to treat a patient with strep throat, a medical professional is not going to go online to search a parent blog for how their child was treated when they had strep throat (hopefully not, at least), but will use any number of vetted reliable references for finding the established dose based upon age, weight, and condition. Unfortunately, nonmedical professionals may not appreciate the difference in quality of information obtained from various sites.

Celebrities, popular blogs, and alternative medicine practitioners with large followings often provide specific medical information that draws attention away from less popular but properly trained medical professionals. Search engine algorithms also link to non-evidence-based sources of information. Thus, when someone without medical experience searches online for medical information, they must be able to identify non-evidence-based sources (not easy), recognize the significant difference between anecdotes and evidence (a pervasive challenge), and appreciate that the opinion of a nonmedically trained celebrity has no comparison to that of a trained medical expert (good luck – we aren't nearly as charismatic or good-looking). On top of all that noise, there are countless sites that provide medical information while also selling their own products or services, which is a huge conflict of interest. The sheer volume of information available online makes it impossible for this arena to ever be regulated or vetted in any reliable manner. A valuable role for medical professionals is to help teach our patients about these pitfalls and how to identify and avoid some common areas of misinformation.

In an effort to better understand how our patients and colleagues are being led astray through misinformation encountered online, try searching online from the patient perspective. It is a valuable exercise to spend time searching common terms or conditions to see the various sites that appear through search engines. Pay attention to the tremendous volume of information and also the more popular sites and links associated with each topic or search term. Then, once you've reached an adequate level of frustration, take the same approach on social media. Social media, particularly Twitter, can offer tremendous insight for medical professionals in regard to the information their patients are receiving not only online but from friends and relatives as well. This knowledge and understanding is useful not only in formulating Twitter posts or articles to combat misinformation but in personal clinical encounters. This type of insight offers the savvy medical professional a peek behind the curtain and helps them appreciate how their patients are thinking through their diagnosis and treatment. You may feel confident in suggesting a proven, evidence-based treatment to your patient, but they may have spent weeks searching through alternative medicine sites and discussing with patients who anecdotally report success through unproven methods in social media circles.

Another useful exercise is to search for the same medical topic in two different places: Google and PubMed. You will often find that the same exact search (assuming proper search terms are used) will yield vastly different results from these two sources. For instance, searching "artificial red dye allergy" (a frequently reported allergy which doesn't actually exist) on Google yields four million results, whereas the same search on PubMed yields 3 results, and only 1 of them is relevant. Try this with various conditions and questions, and you will quickly learn of the tremendous disparities in quality of information. An interesting sidebar to my foray into myth busting is the lack of evidence, particularly high-quality evidence, that supports much of what we routinely do in medicine. This is another valuable exercise: spending time searching for evidence supporting common testing or treatment options for various conditions.

The Choosing Wisely campaign was created by the American Board of Internal Medicine in 2012 [4]. In conjunction with over 70 medical specialties, the Choosing Wisely campaign has identified common tests and treatments that are routinely overused. In addition to a website, Choosing Wisely has free, easy to print posters that can be hung in offices or patient care areas. These lists clearly identify common areas of over testing or overtreatment, provide a brief explanation of why that practice is incorrect, and also list references. This evidence-based approach covers everything from overuse of antibiotics in treating viral upper respiratory infections to need to use spirometry in diagnosing and managing asthma. In addition to providing excellent information and education, the Choosing Wisely campaign is a great source of information for posting to social media. Not only is it important, but it is timely, a source of common misinformation, and vetted by professional organizations.

A fascinating phenomenon is taking place on social media where unqualified individuals are offering specific medical advice to others. Parents routinely post questions or even pictures of their child's rash in Facebook groups asking if anyone has any thoughts [5]. In an effort to help, other parents, regardless of their lack of any medical training whatsoever, offer specific recommendations. There is little consideration that this information may be incorrect, potentially harmful, or lead to delay in proper treatment. There is also little consideration of liability toward the person providing medical recommendations should the information they provide lead to an untoward outcome. But why would parents not just call their child's pediatrician? What leads them to turn to Facebook when their child becomes ill? As a physician, it is terribly disheartening to think that my patients would rather ask anonymous strangers for specific medical advice than call me with their questions. When asked about these behaviors, parents report a myriad of reasons, including a poor relationship with their own physician, lack of trust in the medical establishment, the convenience of posting online at all hours and receiving a reply within minutes, trust in fellow patients or parents who are familiar with their own condition or concerns, and trust in their social media circles, a place where they spend considerable time cultivating relationships.

Twitter 101: How to Engage

As with other social media platforms, Twitter offers some unique features designed to increase engagement. With a 280-character limit, many liken Twitter to micro blogging, where individual tweets can be used to convey ideas, thoughts, and opinions while providing links to longer format articles or websites. There is a bit of a learning curve involved with using Twitter, but with some practice, novice users can become experts rather quickly [6]. Here is a primer for important Twitter concepts and features that medical professionals need to understand:

- Like – Liking a tweet keeps it in your personal list and indicates you appreciate it. This is useful when you want to bookmark an article, research study, or other useful tweets posted by other users as this allows you to easily search your own homepage for tweets that you previously saved to one location for easy recall.
- List – You can create lists of accounts to group together and open a separate timeline. For example, you may wish to create a list for colleagues you follow, one for topics of interest, and one for nonmedical accounts that you follow. This can increase the functionality of Twitter by reducing time spent scrolling through past or recent tweets and focusing the search.
- Mention – Use @ followed by username to "mention" someone else in your tweets. This ensures your tweet will end up in their notifications and timeline. This can increase visibility for those who may not have previously known of your account, can start conversations on a common thread of linked tweets, and can be used to forward tweets from others into a user's account.
- Notifications – This separate timeline displays your interactions with other Twitter users, i.e., mentions, favorites, retweets, and recent followers. This is the area on Twitter where each user should check in on the most regular basis to ensure timely replies to those seeking information or asking questions. This page remains current with the last notification, and users can resume their scrolling where they last logged off or closed their Twitter page.
- Retweet (n.), RT – A tweet you forward to your followers. Can add comments to the original tweet before retweeting. This is how posts get shared with other users on Twitter and ultimately how tweets can go viral.
- Retweet (v.) – The act of sharing another user's tweet to all of your followers.
- Trends – A topic or hashtag determined by algorithms to be the most popular at that moment. Users can set their continuously updated trending topics list to a specific geographic location. Trending topics can include specific hashtags, names of people, or topics.
- Direct messages – Engage in a private conversation with any other Twitter user, as long as they allow for direct messages to be sent to them in their security settings.

These tweets are not seen by anyone other than the two accounts and serve as a manner to take any discussion "offline" while staying on Twitter. This is not a secure method, however, as screenshots of direct messages can easily be obtained and then made public.

Now that we've covered the basics, there are some general principles that can help increase engagement on Twitter. First, interact! If you are merely posting your own Tweets and never replying, thanking others for their retweets/comments, or retweeting content from others, then your account will be viewed as less valuable and sterile. A simple response is all that is necessary most of the time, but it demonstrates your interest in engagement. It can also help to post encouraging messages in general, or to others. For instance, at the start of flu season, you could post a Tweet such as "Flu season is upon us, but we can all stay as healthy as possible by getting our flu vaccine, avoiding close contact with others who are sick, consistently washing our hands, exercising regularly, and getting a good night's sleep." Simple, yet informative and encouraging.

As a medical professional, you will inevitably receive questions on Twitter. This is a great opportunity to engage with others. While you may not be able to offer specific medical advice, you can still reply in a timely fashion and provide a link to general information related to their question. Remember – even if you are interacting with only one other person at a time, anyone who visits your timeline can observe your tweets and replies. Others will see how you engage with those who ask questions, and this can influence their desire to interact with you as well. If you ignore questions/comments or reply in a rude manner, this will also be observed and can negatively impact your online reputation. You can always take it offline or interact through direct messaging as well. Chapter 10 offers a much more thorough discussion of how to deal with trolls or those who purposefully try to elicit an emotional or argumentative reply.

Take Advantage of Trending Topics

The concept of trending topics was introduced earlier in this chapter. Each day, there will be various topics or hashtags that will be listed as trending by Twitter. This often revolves around popular media stories, late breaking news, celebrities, or popular sporting events. If a topic is trending that relates to your area of interest, you can join the conversation or post information using that hashtag to help increase engagement. CAUTION: Always scroll through the tweets associated with the trending topic or hashtag before you post yourself! There are interesting examples of hashtags seeming straightforward but are completely unrelated and can include inappropriate content. Trends are determined by an algorithm and tailored according to followers, interests, and location. The algorithm is designed to identify popular topics at that moment, not in the days or weeks prior, which makes this feature a method for staying as current as possible.

When you click on a trending topic or hashtag, you are taken to the Twitter search results for that trend. From there, or from your own homepage/timeline, you can easily participate in a trend by simply posting a tweet with the exact same word, phrase, or hashtag that appears in the trend. In general, Twitter prevents topics promoting adult references, discrimination, or hate content from trending. But difficult subject matter is not off limits, including tragic events or loss of life. As you gain practice with Twitter and trending hashtags, you will encounter examples of accounts that use tragedy to promote their account or sell their product. As discussed previously in this textbook, many people use Twitter as their main source of information, and media outlets all report late breaking news through their Twitter feeds. As such, when tragic events such as natural disasters, terrorist attacks, or deaths of prominent individuals occur, they will start trending. This is not the opportunity medical professionals should use to capitalize on a popular hashtag or topic. It takes years of consistency to build trust with your followers, and that can all disappear with ill-timed or intentioned tweets.

The Twitter settings feature allows each account to set and change the way their trends are displayed. You can choose to have trends from across the United States be featured or your specific location (Fig. 6.3). This will change the trending topics that appear on your homepage, thus it is important to understand these differences.

As a medical professional, you will need to decide if you want to maintain a pure professional presence on social media, a personal presence, or a mixture of both.

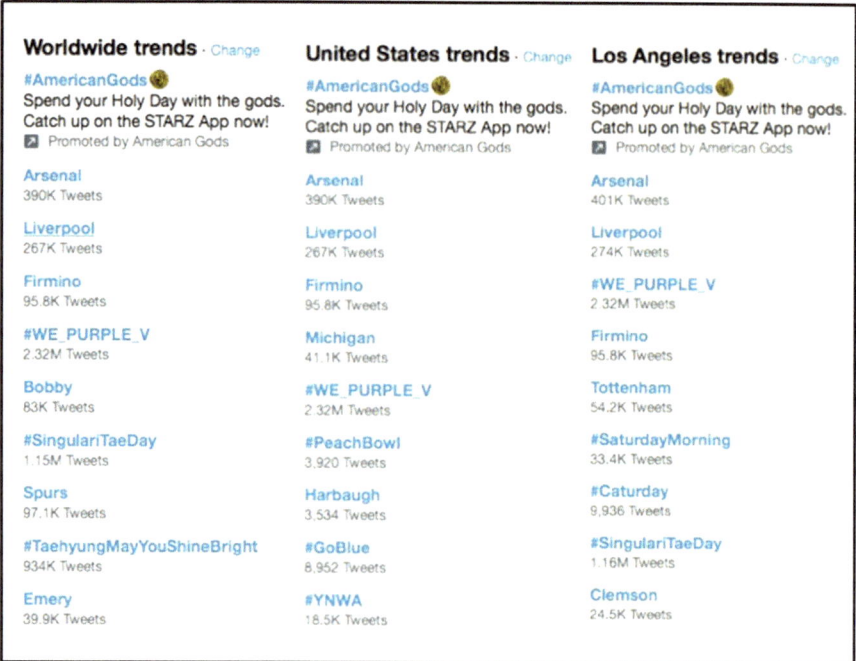

Fig. 6.3 Trending topics vary by location

Personally, I have melded by role as a pediatric allergist with my experience as a father and a husband and with some of my personal interests. I also allow my sense of humor to be portrayed in various ways. This was a conscious decision and one I felt comfortable making, but this approach is not suited for everyone. Regardless, humorous trending topics can be incorporated with medical information in unique and creative ways. Here are a few examples of how I utilized popular trending topics to disseminate medical information (Fig. 6.4).

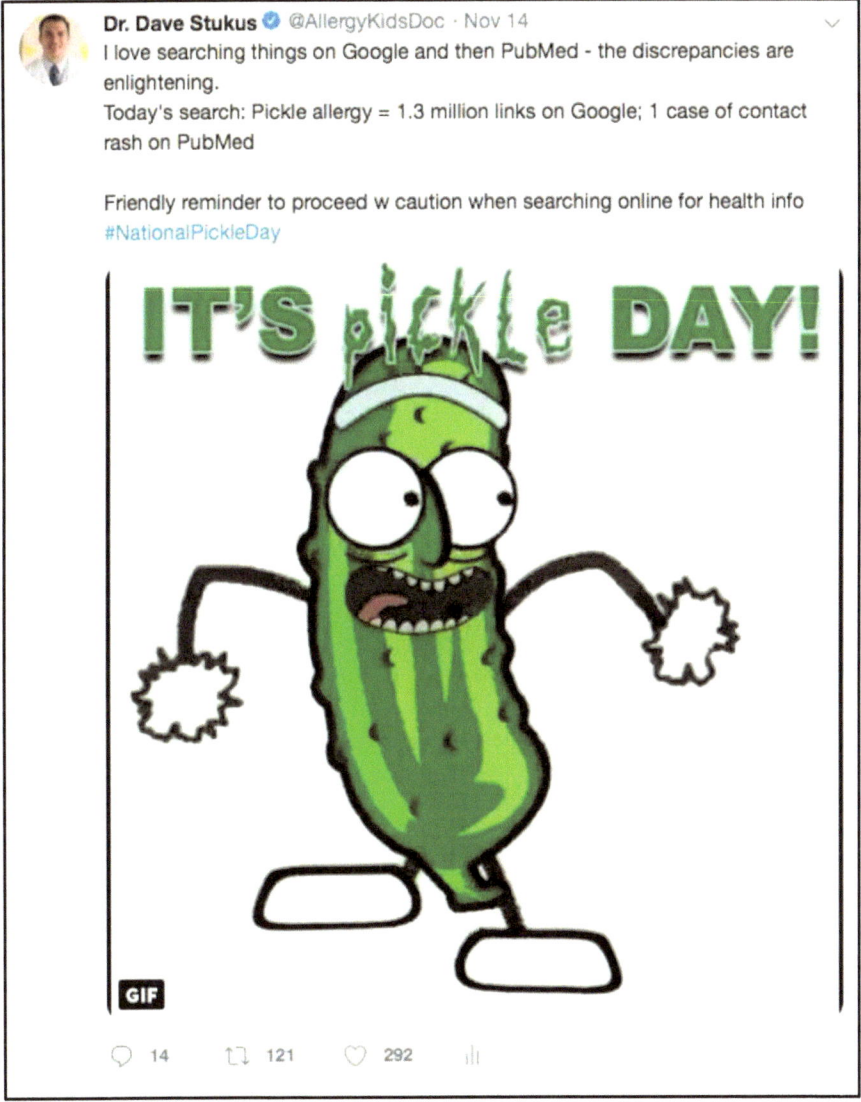

Fig. 6.4 Examples of using nonmedical trending topics to disseminate medical information. (Adapted from https://twitter.com/AllergyKidsDoc)

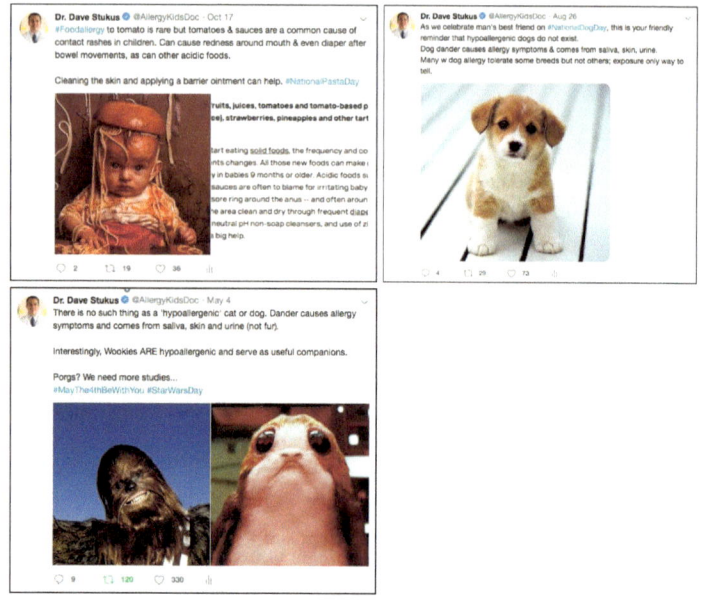

Fig. 6.4 (continued)

Hashtags

A hashtag refers to the symbol "#." When # is placed immediately before any word, phrase, or characters, it allows Twitter to index keywords or topics. This enables users to easily follow, search for, or discover topics they are interested in. One of the easiest ways to grow an audience on Twitter is to discover and utilize relevant hashtags, which will make an account discoverable by anyone searching the same topic. Tweets that incorporate hashtags have twice as much engagement compared with those that have none. Hashtags can be used anywhere within a tweet and, once clicked, will take the user to another page that lists the most popular tweets that also used that hashtag, as well as a chronological listing of all tweets, with the most recent tweets appearing at the top of the page.

In order to be included with all other hashtags in the search, the hashtag cannot be altered in any way, including the addition of spaces, symbols, or punctuation. Twitter allows each post to include as many hashtags as the user desires; however, it is considered poor form to use more than two or three hashtags at most. Each character within a hashtag counts against the 280 character limit as well. Overuse of hashtags within a tweet is viewed by others as spam and less credible – this is akin to receiving unwanted emails from those selling products. Likewise, use of hashtags associated with tragic events or inappropriate material in an effort to increase exposure of a tweet or account is also frowned upon. It is also important to use established hashtags in order to take advantage of the indexing that occurs. Tweets that attempt humor or sarcasm may make up their own hashtag as sort of an inside joke for Twitter users, but this will not make their tweet more discoverable or increase engagement.

As with trending topics, it is important to click through any hashtag before using it in a tweet. Some acronyms, phrases, or topics may have multiple meanings, including inappropriate content. The last thing you or any medical professional wants is to have their tweet inadvertently end up in the same list as inappropriate content! Similar to location impacting the trending topics at any given time, hashtags can be used to reach targeted groups or local communities or join worldwide conversations. In addition, popular topics often have multiple hashtags associated with them, but not all with have the same engagement and reach. Examples include #Christmas #MerryChristmas #Christmas2018, all of which were popular leading up to and on December 25, 2018, but each led to different indices and audiences. You can click on each hashtag to get a sense of number of tweets associated with each one by looking at the latest tweets; if there are no recent posts, then that hashtag is not likely going to generate much engagement. In addition, subtle differences in hashtags can be associated with very different audiences. For example, if you are posting information related to headaches, there are multiple different hashtags that could be included, such as #headache, #migraine, #pain, or even #head. As Fig. 6.5 illustrates, these minor differences are associated with different types of accounts and users.

There are two additional ways that medical professionals can use hashtags to easily and significantly increase their audience. As discussed previously, medical conferences almost universally will announce and use an official hashtag during the meeting. This often includes the acronym for the professional organization followed by the year. All tweets from the meeting will be indexed with each other when using the common hashtag. Sending tweets that include the meeting hashtag

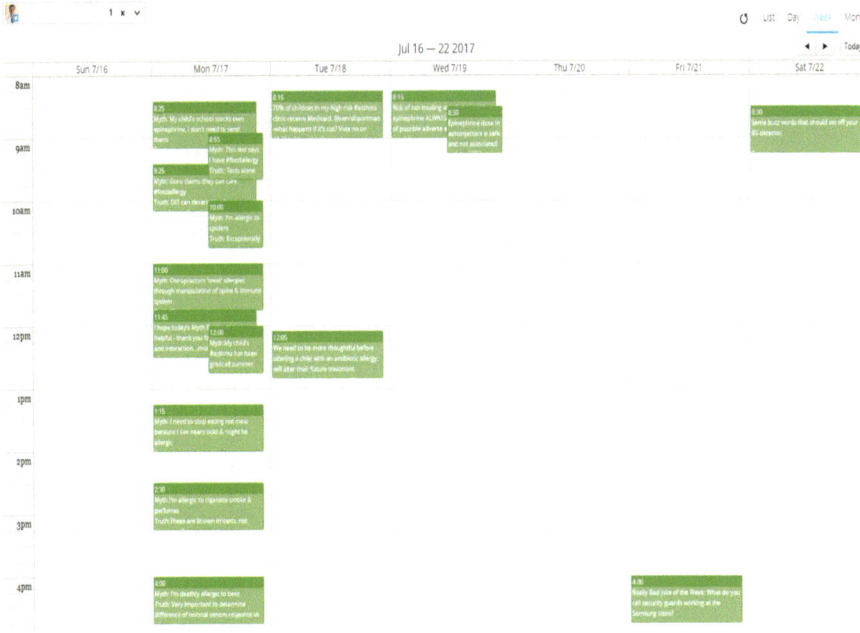

Fig. 6.5 Different hashtags related to the same topic can result in different results

from within sessions, after sessions, or in general while attending the meeting will increase visibility and can also lead to networking with colleagues.

Additionally, live Twitter chats are frequently conducted by professional organizations, medical journals (including virtual journal clubs), advocacy groups, or health-related social media groups. These Twitter chats are announced in advance so everyone knows what time they will occur to maximize participation. The "host" will send out topics every 5–15 minutes, and then participants can post replies or comments. The use of a common hashtag during the live Twitter chat enables participants to follow along, see all associated tweets, and allows anyone to follow along, even if they don't participate. Lastly, the content and discussion during live Twitter chats can be searched anytime afterwards by looking at the hashtag used. With practice and familiarity, medical professionals can discover and utilize hashtags with their Tweets in a way to increase engagement.

Time Management

One of the most frequent questions I get asked by medical professionals interested in joining or increasing their use of social media is how much time I spend on this endeavor. This is a valid concern, especially given the increase in addiction to social media and technology in general. Social media should be enjoyable and rewarding, not a burden. There are some simple tips to help make time management with social media more manageable and less burdensome:

1. Turn off all notifications. Unless you enjoy getting a ding or a buzz every time your tweet is retweeted, liked, or replied to, this is the first step everyone should take in order to make social media less intrusive. My personal rule is that I interact with social media on my schedule and when I want to devote attention to it, not the other way around. I have many family members, friends, and colleagues who follow my Twitter account and at times I have received text messages from them regarding my content, or content of others. I have learned to politely ask them to not use text messaging for social media-related concerns as that is intrusive on my personal time. Learning to make social media work for you, and not you working for social media, is a significant step to avoiding social media burn out.
2. Find the pattern that fits with your lifestyle. I am an early riser and typically have 30 minutes each morning to myself before my wife and children wake. I use this early morning time (7–7:30 am) to check my notifications, reply to any questions, and post new content for that day. I will typically not check Twitter again until lunch time and then spend 10–15 minutes catching up. I practice in an outpatient setting and typically finish with my clinical and administrative duties around 4:30 pm and will very quickly check my Twitter feed while I walk to my car. I will then *briefly* check Twitter before bed often while brushing my teeth. I take advantage of the mobile feature on my cellphone and can then check in when I want and when it's convenient. A typical day may include ~60 minutes total on social media but spread out in small increments. This pattern fits my lifestyle and work habits but may not work for someone else. Many

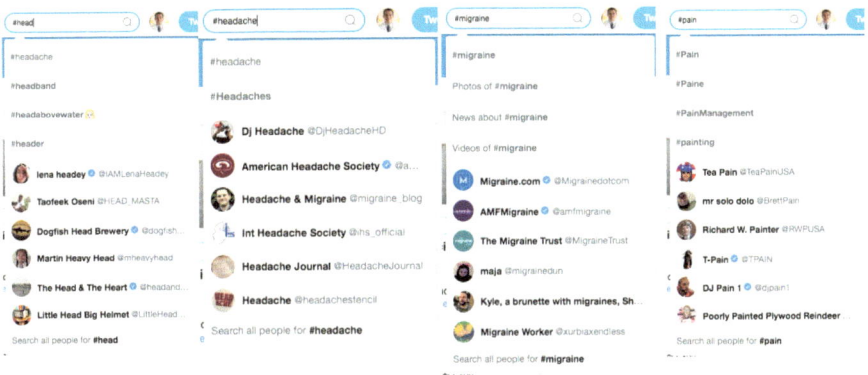

Fig. 6.6 The dashboard from Hootsuite on a busy Myth Buster Monday. (Adapted from https://hootsuite.com)

of my colleagues check their Twitter feed once a day, or every other day, and this works perfectly for them. Unfortunately, others are seemingly on their devices nonstop, often to the detriment of work or personal obligations.

3. Use online schedulers. No one has time to be on Twitter or social media every minute throughout the day. As one's platform and audience grows, followers from around the world will appear and participate in engagement. This means different time zones and different patterns of utilization among one's followers. One way to not only manage one's own time more effectively and reach followers in various time zones is to use any number of social media scheduling services, many of which are available for free. Scheduling tweets allows users to plan their online campaign and arrange for ongoing posts during vacation or time away from social media and removes the worry of trying to find time to post tweets during busy periods at work or home. Hootsuite, Tweetdeck, and Buffer are a few platforms that allow users to schedule Tweets at any time. See Fig. 6.6 for an example of how I schedule a busy Myth Buster Monday full of tweets before heading off to work.

4. Don't set it and forget it. If you choose to use an online scheduler, be mindful of two important aspects. First, if a tragic event occurs or online discussion is trending toward a very serious matter, make sure that you don't have any tweets scheduled at that time. For instance, it will be poor form to have humorous tweets scheduled to be sent out shortly after a terrorist attack or natural disaster occurs. Second, it is important to check in periodically in case another user has questions or comments on one of your scheduled tweets.

Use Metrics to Increase Engagement

Twitter incorporates detailed analytics for each account, which are easily accessible and available for review at any time. This is a useful tool that offers data for better understanding which tweets generated the most engagement and interest. This can be used to understand how one's audience engages in regard to content, day of the week, time of day, and part of each month. For instance, I learned that tweets I post early in the morning on Mondays and Tuesdays typically generate far more interest than tweets sent on Thursday or Friday mornings, or in the afternoon. This likely relates to my large number of followers who are also medical professionals who have similar habits as myself. With this knowledge, I will often save more useful or important information for the times when engagement will likely be highest. However, I will still experiment and retweet my own posts at various times throughout the week, particularly if something generates interest among my followers. Keep in mind that as your audience grows, it will change as well. It helps to periodically monitor your analytics and try to understand the social media habits and interests of your followers. Figure 6.7 offers examples of the myriad of data available through Twitter.

The terminology utilized by Twitter analytics can seem confusing at first. Table 6.2 offers a guide to better understand these terms.

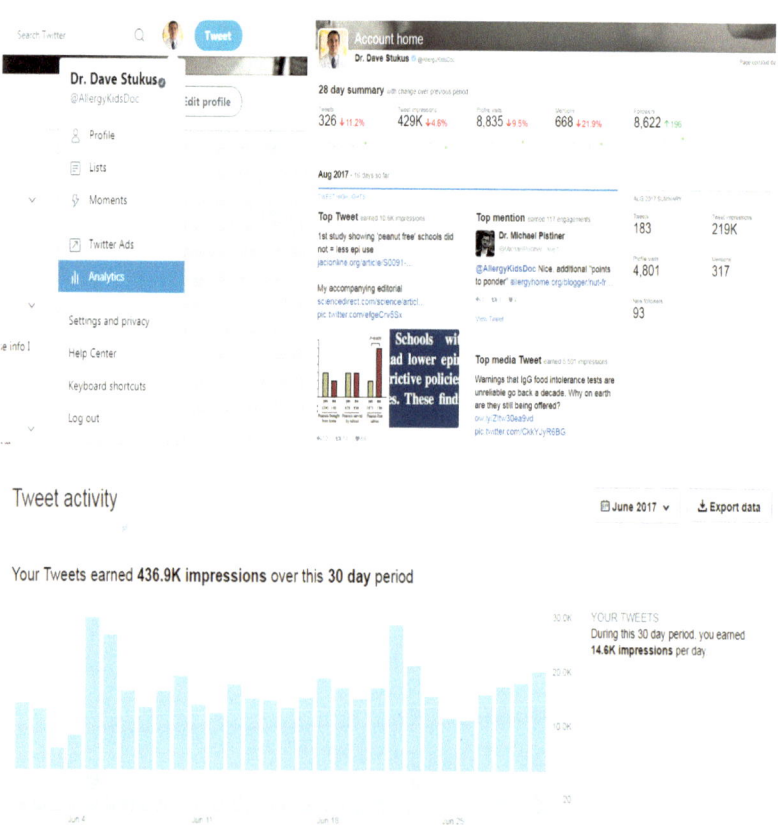

Fig. 6.7   Twitter analytics offer data to help understand engagement. (Adapted from https://twitter.com/AllergyKidsDoc)

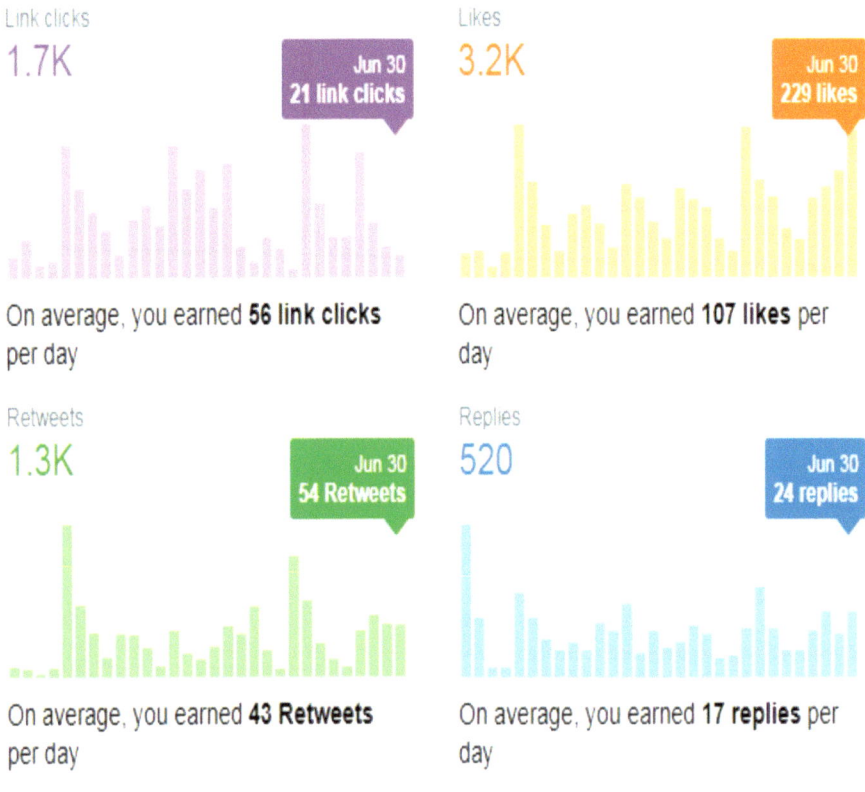

On average, you earned **56 link clicks** per day

On average, you earned **107 likes** per day

On average, you earned **43 Retweets** per day

On average, you earned **17 replies** per day

Fig. 6.7 (continued)

Table 6.2 Terminology used in Twitter analytics

Impressions	Number of times users saw the tweet on Twitter
Engagements	Total number of times a user has interacted with a tweet. This includes clicks anywhere on the tweet (hashtags, links, avatar, username), retweets, replies, follows, and likes
Engagement rate	The number of engagements divided by the total number of impressions
Profile clicks	Number of clicks on the username, @handle, or profile photo

Medical professionals who use Twitter to disseminate information and interact with others can take advantage of these analytic tools to better understand what information and approach garners the widest appeal. More importantly, this data offers positive feedback and reinforcement to support one's efforts. It is amazing to see how one tweet (which costs nothing, by the way) can be seen by hundreds or thousands of people from around the world. Medical professionals can use this data with their administrators to demonstrate their impact, particularly with number of profile clicks. If one links to their practice or hospital in their profile, this amounts to additional advertising. As one's audience grows, the clicks increase, and the impact widens. This can all be demonstrated by collecting and sharing the data offered through Twitter.

Conclusions

As this chapter discussed in detail, Twitter is a very useful social media platform for medical professionals to utilize. As with any social media site, there is a bit of a learning curve for new users in regard to terminology and functionality. By practicing with and using hashtags and trending topics, medical professionals can increase their engagement more rapidly and on a wider scale. As with all other social media channels, Twitter users should always keep in mind the "social" aspect of their account. By taking the time to establish a professional-appearing homepage, background photo, personal photo, and profile, medical professionals can establish themselves as a useful and trusted resource for other Twitter users who find their account.

References

1. www.33charts.com. Last accessed: 20 Dec 2018.
2. https://33charts.com/build-it/. Last accessed: 20 Dec 2018.
3. Morris ZS, Wooding S, Grant J. The answer is 17 years, what is the question: understanding time lags in translational research. J R Soc Med. 2011;104(12):510–20.
4. www.choosingwisely.org. Last accessed: 30 Dec 2018.
5. https://www.kevinmd.com/blog/2013/07/facebook-medical-advice-child.html. Last accessed: 30 Dec 2018.
6. https://help.twitter.com/en/twitter-guide. Last accessed: 30 Dec 2018.

Content Curation

7

How to Identify and Use Information from Credible Sources

Kathryn E. Nuss

If you have knowledge, let others light their candle in it.

—Margaret Fuller

Most of us remember a time before smartphones, iPads, and social media. We grew up using encyclopedias instead of search engines and got our news from the television or newspaper instead of our social feeds. The times have changed, and with those changes, come significant shifts in how healthcare professionals relate to their patients, spread the word about their business, and connect with colleagues in their field. It has changed how patients gain new information about medicine and health, how they choose their healthcare providers, and how they make informed decisions about their medical care.

On a daily basis, about 2 billion people log into Facebook around the world [1]. About 500 million people scroll through Instagram [2]. 335 million log into their Twitter accounts [3]. Every day, millions of people pose questions to their communities, read about the world around them, and read about topics that interest them. According to the Division of Biomedical Informatics at the University of California San Diego, the proportion of adults using social media in the United States increased from 8% in 2005 to 72% in 2014 [4]. Our latest statistics in 2018 indicate that 77% of adults in the United States now use social media [5]. Social media is here to stay, and we very well may see numbers continue to rise as we head into the future.

If you're a physician or healthcare professional, you have probably seen how social media has changed the medical field. Maybe you have even participated in this change yourself. Since the inception of social media, healthcare professionals have used social media sites such as Twitter and Facebook to share information and to promote health behaviors among their patients and to spread knowledge about their practice and its daily operations to the general public. They've used social media to provide health information to their communities, to share research ideas

© Springer Nature Switzerland AG 2019 121
D. R. Stukus et al., *Social Media for Medical Professionals*,
https://doi.org/10.1007/978-3-030-14439-5_7

with other physicians, and to even augment clinical care by communicating directly with patients and caregivers [6, 7].

But while the use of social media by healthcare professionals can help doctors, patients, and practices, the misuse of social media can destroy the public's trust in a practice or practitioner and can damage a physician or hospital's reputation. Furthermore, the healthcare professional who seeks to augment their practice over social media should be aware of how time-consuming it can be to create their own content and how much time and energy it takes to form a loyal online following. This chapter will discuss the best ways to curate content, why a healthcare professional should curate content as opposed to creating regular content themselves, and perhaps most importantly, how they can find content that's trustworthy and reliable and will improve their professional reputation – not harm it.

Social Media as a Pipeline to Knowledge

For better or worse, social media is increasingly being used as a primary information source for many Americans, whether for news or health information. A 2016 survey [8] by Health Union reports that 65% of patients use Facebook for health information. A Pew Research Poll conducted a year later maintained that 67% of Americans get their news at least in part through social media [9].

Mothers especially tend to log onto their favorite social network such as Twitter or Facebook in order to ask their support group for information. Often, mothers ask questions about their child's health, turning to social media platforms to discuss health concerns, home remedies, and to even diagnose their children. According to a Pew Research study [10] from 2015, 71% of parents on social media try to respond if they know (or think they know) the answer to a question posed by someone in their online network. Furthermore, 79% of parents agree that they get useful information through their social media networks. Fifty nine percent claim that they've come across useful information specifically about parenting in the last 30 days while looking at other social media content. According to the poll, mothers are particularly likely to encounter helpful parenting information. One can only wonder if these numbers have inched up throughout the years since 2015, as more and more parents log on and as more digital natives have children.

"I love that moms are connecting on social media," says Wendy Sue Swanson, MD, chief of digital innovation at Seattle Children's Hospital and author of the blog Seattle Mama Doc, "But you don't want to confuse experience with expertise." [11]

You'd think that Americans would be pretty good at avoiding misinformation by now. Studies show that Americans and westerners in general hold analytical and logical approaches to information seeking. Americans have been told over and over again that we need to vet what we find online and that we can't trust everything we read on the Internet. But inevitably, mothers end up listening to the aunt in Phoenix who thinks she knows a thing or two about colic or the old friend from high school with health theories of her own.

This is true for patients with chronic conditions as well. While on social media, people can easily and efficiently find other people who have the same health experiences and concerns. Social media is full of support groups for cancer patients, people with lupus, people with rheumatoid arthritis, and any other health condition you could possibly think of. A 2010 report [12] by the Pew Internet & American Life Project found that more than half of patients living with chronic disease are avid consumers of user-generated health information on social media. These patients read the commentaries of others who are struggling with the same chronic illness, they read about health and medical issues in forums, websites, and blogs, and they share information, emotional support, and practical advice.

One in five patients living with chronic disease creates online health content. They write blogs, post comments, and share information about health and medical matters in an online group forum or discussion. While this is a wonderful support opportunity, it might not always be the best place for our patients to find accurate health information.

One e-patient wrote to Pew Research, "I spend a lot of time looking for information on the internet. It has been an invaluable resource for me. In addition, I keep a blog so that I can keep all my information in one place. Having a rare disorder along with chronic pain, I need all the help I can get – but I do great. I have a full time job, and participate in many activities, including a half marathon in May – and many of the things I have learned have been from the internet." Clearly, the search for information online can give patients a deeper sense of understanding and control over their health and can foster online communities of people who struggle with the same health issues.

The good news is that studies indicate that expertise-based health information sites are used more frequently (and trusted more) by Americans. Sites such as MedlinePlus, the Mayo Clinic, WebMD, Healthline Networks, and the Centers for Disease Control and Prevention are top sites that are trusted by the majority of American patients. While there's plenty of false information out there, Americans at least try to gather their information from sites they can trust. But make no mistake, the amount of false or misleading information on social media is still a public health problem.

At its best, social media can be a good thing for patients because it can increase access to health information and improve a patient's understanding of a health issue. Informed patients [13] receive higher-quality care because they understand their options and share essential information with their healthcare providers. Informed patients are clear about their health goals and are an active part in the decision-making process around their own healthcare.

Healthcare professionals can leverage social media as a way to share quality health information and to create more informed patients. Healthcare professionals can disseminate expertise-based health information online, which enhances a patient's access to that information and allows the patient to understand how the information is relevant to them, and, since it's coming from a doctor, the patient is likely to consider the information credible [14].

Finding Credible Sources About Healthcare on the Internet Can Be Difficult

Many healthcare professionals have to counsel worried patients who come into their practice sharing incredible theories and concerns about something they read online. It's actually become somewhat of a joke among internet users, "Whatever symptoms you have, don't look them up online!" What begins as a harmless headache can quickly snowball into anxiety about a brain tumor if a patient tries to diagnose themselves online. Many doctors squelch patient concerns about whether hormonal birth control will give them breast cancer or whether a child's vaccine will result in autism. Perhaps it's good that it creates more conversation between patients and doctors, but we cannot be sure as to what these information sources do to a patient's understanding and trust in their doctors.

The internet is the wild, wild west. There are very few rules. Someone can publish an official-looking article that claims that all western medicine is evil (and someone probably has).

While many patients have gotten skilled at discerning credible vs. non-credible information, bias sneaks in, information is incomplete, sources are unreferenced, and our patients end up with sub-par information. Social media users might not be able to recognize hidden bias or either hidden or overt conflicts of interest that renders the information questionable.

The rise of social media means that medical professionals are no longer the only source of healthcare information. Now, the control of medical knowledge is shifting from trained and expert health professionals to the larger social community [15]. A young mother with an opinion might garner a large following and be considered a reliable source of health and medical information. This is why it's essential for healthcare professionals to join in on the conversation.

Furthermore, information found online often lacks the professional gatekeepers to check the validity of content [16]. We now lack the traditional markers used to determine whether a source is credible or not. This means that now patients are more responsible than ever when it comes to discerning whether an online source is credible. A source that one patient considers credible, another might scoff at for its lack of credibility and trustworthiness. Patients may have a difficult time agreeing which information is accurate and which is not.

There are also plenty of organizations that spread misinformation because they're trying to push a certain belief. They tweak the information to fit a certain perspective. Special interest blogs and websites might cite accurate studies but then interpret that information in a way that benefits their perspective. This can lead to a misunderstanding of a study's findings, and some social media users won't be able to tell the difference between accurate and biased content.

There are a lot of voices on the internet. Every single day, 3.7 billion humans access the World Wide Web. Every day, there are 3.5 billion google searches performed and 456,000 tweets. Many Internet users aren't sure how to wade through all the hype, clickbait, and nonsensical information about health. In fact, misinformation on the internet was cited by 50 experts interviewed by the BBC as one of the "grand challenges we face in the 21st century" [17]. We find ourselves in a situation where "objective facts are less influential in shaping public opinion than appeals to emotion and personal belief." [18]

According to Kevin Kelly, co-founder of *Wired* Magazine, "Truth is no longer dictated by authorities, but is networked by peers. For every fact there is a counter-fact and all these counterfacts and facts look identical online, which is confusing to most people." So in this day-in-age where people can find bogus health information, and where bogus health "false facts" are just as easy to find – if not easier – than actual medical truths, it's more essential than ever to be diligent on where we pull our information.

Dr. Brittany Seymour, assistant professor of oral health policy and epidemiology at Harvard University, cites the public vaccine scare as a prime example of misinformation online threatening public health. In 2014, the United States had one of the largest measles outbreaks in a generation. "We've been able to trace that, in part, to parents who found scary information on the internet and opted to not vaccinate their children." [19]

The balance of influence has shifted. Now, the informing power is in the hands of the individual with a smartphone and a Twitter account. Among all the misinformation, it's more essential than ever to cite evidence-based information. It's essential to know *how* to find accurate information, how to discern between fake and fact, and what it means to be credible.

What It Means to Be Credible

Studies show that certain behaviors affect someone's perceived credibility online [16]. Readers, whether consciously or not, decide whether the writer (or sharer of information) knows the truth. They decide whether they believe the writer or sharer will tell the truth as they know it. They decide whether the writer has the best interests of the reader at heart.

When people read information online, they factor the credentials of the author when it comes to gauging trustworthiness. (Does this author know what they're talking about? Are they an expert? Are they a professional in the field in which they're spreading information?) For example, authors with medical credentials are perceived as having higher levels of expertise, and their information is perceived as more credible.

Perhaps more surprisingly, readers negatively perceive language that is overly technical. If an author uses overly technical language, filled with jargon and fancy words, the reader is less likely to view the source as credible. (Maybe this is because readers perceive these authors as trying too hard? Or perhaps they perceive these authors as having less of a grasp on the concept they're trying to convey) [20]. So be sure to speak to your audience.

As physicians, pharmacists, and other healthcare professionals, we have a leg up when it comes to credibility. Some studies suggest that patients trust their doctors more than what they might find in an internet search. A 2010 study [21] shows that when doctor-patient communications are strong, people are less likely to look for alternative health resources online. In another study [22] on American seniors, they found that people are more likely to depend on face-to-face interactions with their doctors and pharmacists over gaining health information online. When doctors log on, they have a critical responsibility to share only the most accurate information from the most credible sources.

So how can doctors ensure they share only credible information? According to the University of California San Francisco [23], there are a few ways to correctly evaluate health information online:

1. The article in question has an identifiable source or author.
2. The particular source is likely to be fair, objective, and lacking in hidden motives.
3. The author has the credentials or the required expertise and training to provide the information (for medical information, it's best to source from a medical institution, a government health agency, or a medically knowledgeable professional).
4. The publication has undergone peer review by a panel of professionals in the field.

Finding accurate information goes a little deeper than mere credibility. Even if you're identified as a credible source, it's essential to dig deeper to discern whether the information itself can be trusted. The University of California at San Francisco also gives us a clear roadmap on how to tell if the information itself may be accurate:

1. The information is supported by evidence from scientific studies, other data, or expert opinion.
2. The information is based on a large sample or comes from randomized, controlled studies.
3. The authors discuss any limitations or weaknesses of the study.

Sometimes, the healthcare professional on Twitter might choose to share information from a secondary source, such as a newspaper article. This is fine, but keep in mind that articles such as these are coming from a writer's interpretation of the data. In such cases, a writer's opinion might get in the way of their ability to accurately represent the studies she is citing.

Credibility Red Flags

How can we tell whether the information at hand is trustworthy? How do we know when to walk away, so to speak, from a less-than-ideal publication, article, study, or piece of content? Here are some warning signs that will tell you that a piece of content isn't worth your time:

1. The author remains anonymous.
2. There is a conflict of interest.
3. The information appears to be biased or one-sided.

For example, Dr. Vinay Prasad [24] from Portland Oregon says, "I see doctors tweeting about cancer drugs who were only giving the upside to drugs I knew were not necessarily the safest or most affordable option. When I would bring this up, they would tweet "It's not a problem" or "It's not a concern." I'd then look them up, and they usually had a financial conflict of interest. So they're tweeting about drugs and not telling people they get money."

4. The information is outdated (typically we don't want to rely on medical information that's more than 3 years old).
5. There is a claim of a miracle or secret cure.
6. No evidence is cited.
7. Grammar is poor and words are misspelled.

It's best to stay clear from sources with these red flags. Our job as healthcare professionals is to help spread accurate health information to empower our patients. If we don't critically examine each source we curate, we might end up misinforming followers and losing the trust of others.

This is Why It's Essential for Healthcare Professionals to be Smart Online!

There's no doubt that healthcare professionals have a huge responsibility in their practices, but they also have a huge responsibility when they go online. Everything we post – whether on our professional or personal social media accounts – impacts the trust of our patients and potentially their health outcomes.

On social media, the presence of healthcare professionals can serve as a torch in the dark. While there are plenty of bogus sites out there and as misinformation circulates around our patients, we can light the way for our patients who want to become more knowledgeable about health and medicine. Healthcare professionals on social media can, and should, serve as beacons of truth when it comes to educating the public. Every healthcare professional who uses social media to spread health information serves as an antidote to nonsense in the social media world.

The presence of physicians on social media has already changed the way that patients relate to doctors. Now, patients don't have to wait until their next appointment in order to find answers to their questions. Our patients can now easily access medical information from the healthcare professionals they trust. What's more, social media users are more likely to trust information given by their local doctors. They may perceive the information their doctors give as more relevant. It's coming from a source that's "close to home."

In fact, 60% of social media users are more likely to trust social media posts by physicians over any other group [25]. Healthcare organizations such as hospitals and private practices understand this. More and more leading healthcare organizations are building their social media sites, offering their consumers health information right where they can easily access it.

How Using Social Media Can Help Healthcare Professionals

Chances are, if you're reading this, you're a doctor or healthcare professional. You know that healthcare providers do not have an abundance of time. The reluctant practitioner might ask, "But why *should* healthcare professionals use social media? Sure, we can educate our patients. We can help spread the right information. But what's in it for the healthcare professional?"

The arrival of social media has significantly changed the networking landscape for all professionals, including doctors. Social media connects doctors, allowing them to discuss challenges in their respective field or specialty. In this day-in-age of increasing focus among healthcare professionals, it can be difficult to find other doctors who specialize in what you specialize in and who understand the same trials and challenges of that specialty. A highly specialized physician in Cleveland can connect with a similar specialist in Maryland. Through social media, they can discuss unique challenges in their field of medicine.

And just as social media is a pipeline of knowledge for patients, it can serve the same purpose for doctors. Physicians join online communities where they can become more informed and access new information. A doctor's social media feed can be a central hub for new research, news articles, expert opinions, and medical developments. Social media can be a time-effective way to stay up to date on medical tech, new treatment options, and new developments in the field.

Finally, a healthcare professional joining social media enhances the visibility of her organization. Providers who have an active following on social media catapult their organizations into the spotlight, giving that practice or organization credibility, visibility, and a social perception of being "cutting-edge." Doctors use social media to grow their practice, to fundraise, to improve customer service and support, to educate patients, and to advertise new services [7].

In fact, using social media is just good marketing for your practice or hospital. Studies show that healthcare organizations regularly benefit from logging into social media sites. Twelve and a half percent of surveyed healthcare organizations reported having successfully attracted new patients through the use of social media. When medical centers, doctor's offices, and hospitals use social media correctly, their visibility and image is enhanced.

In one study, 57% of consumers said that a hospital's social media presence strongly influences their choice of where to go for services. Why? Patients like being able to see the quality of facilities where their care will take place. A hospital with a strong social media presence is interpreted by patients as being an indication that the hospital offers cutting-edge or state-of-the-art technologies [26].

This boost in image can be said for individual doctors as well. Doctors who create a healthy social media presence can end up with thousands of followers. Through their social media, these doctors become thought leaders and well-known industry experts. Many doctors that I mention toward the end of this chapter have seen incredible benefits to their careers with the help of their social media work. They've been invited to speak at conferences, to give Ted Talks, to write books, and to share their professional opinions in national discussions about health and disease.

How Social Media Helps Patients

It's no wonder the era in which we live is constantly referred to as "the information age." Patients can perform their own health research online from something they saw on social media. On Twitter, 59.9% of patients log on to increase their knowledge and to exchange advice with others. On Facebook, 52.3% of patients seek social support around health issues and seek advice for medical concerns [27].

Through social media, patients can learn about healthy habits, especially when they're following healthcare professionals and organizations. They can easily and effortlessly obtain relevant health and medical information that makes sense to them. Patients can easily attain important information about health through their physicians or other doctors on the internet.

This increased knowledge about health leads to increased patient empowerment. Social networks help support sound decision-making, and patients are now taking the reins when it comes to engaging in their own health efforts, setting health goals, and tracking their own health progress [28]. Never before have patients been able to discuss and research their personal health concerns with so much support as now in the social media age.

Social media is also helping patients create crowd support [29]. Many patients, especially those living with chronic health conditions and disabilities, find emotional (and even financial) support from within their chosen online groups and communities.

It's even better when a patient's doctor is on social media to help guide and educate them. Especially in an online climate where not all information can be trusted, healthcare professionals can guide patients to credible peer-reviewed websites where the information is subject to quality control [30]. Through social media, doctors can provide information and tools to their patients, promote healthy behaviors, and engage with their patients, students, and colleagues.

Healthcare professionals logging onto social media may also improve patient trust. Studies show that patient trust in physicians has declined sharply over the past half century. In 1966, 73% of Americans said they had "great confidence in the leaders of the medical profession." In 2012, only 34% of Americans expressed this view [31].

Studies show that in order to win back patient trust, being more communicative and open with our patients is essential. Typically, Americans are highly trusting of their own doctors but weary of the healthcare system as a whole. Doctors who log onto social media can increase patient trust by visibly taking a stance that would improve the nation's healthcare. Doctors can show patients that they put the needs of the patient first. According to a 2004 study [32], healthcare professionals can achieve patient trust by:

1. Showing their patients that they share a mutual interest in the patient's health
2. Clearly communicating
3. Repeatedly fulfilling patient trust
4. Reducing power differences by sharing information
5. Responding to what their patients tell them in an accepting and nonjudgmental way
6. Promoting a long-term doctor-patient relationship

A doctor who logs onto social media can achieve most, if not all, of these behaviors that earn trust. They can share information online that shows their interest in positive patient outcomes, they can communicate more clearly with patients and caregivers, and they can share information that levels the playing field.

Studies show that patients who trust their healthcare professionals are more likely to follow treatment plans, therefore experiencing more favorable health outcomes. Patients who do not trust their providers are less likely to seek treatment in the first place.

Who Are You Online?

With a thorough understanding of how social media can help both healthcare professionals and patients, providers can take the first step in assuring an utmost professional online presence by asking themselves a single question: "Who am I online?"

When professionals use social media, they're not just representing themselves as individuals – they're representing their practice, hospital, or organization. They're representing all of healthcare as a whole. How healthcare professionals convey themselves over social media can significantly inform – and destroy – a patient's trust in them.

First, think about the type of content you will share. You should have one overarching theme and about two to three sub-themes. These themes will tell the world what you care about, what you stand for, and how you can help your readers.

For example, if you're a neuroscientist who specializes in Alzheimer's care, your overarching theme will be the neuroscience around Alzheimer's disease. Your subthemes could include brain-healthy nutrition, preventative measures, and how caregivers and families can provide the best support possible (see Fig. 7.1). On your social media pages, you can share articles, studies, infographics, stories, and other information that fit within any of these silos.

Topics of discussion can vary widely. You can decide what your social media site is going to focus on – how it's going to represent what you think about as a doctor. You can share clinical topics, ethics concerns, politics around healthcare,

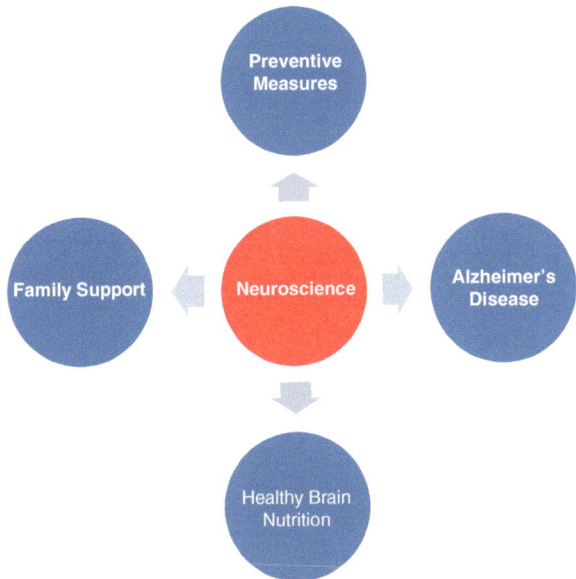

Fig. 7.1 Different content areas can be explored for any topic

statistics, issues around practice management, career strategies for healthcare professionals, and just about anything else you can think of that might resonate with your audience.

Speaking of an audience, you have to know who you're talking to. It can sometimes feel like you're talking to a wall when you send your first couple of tweets, but it's best to start with a full understanding of who your target audience is and what they care about. (For example, if your audience is pediatric oncologists, posts about horse racing in Kentucky might feel irrelevant to them.)

Perhaps most importantly to the health of your career and practice, consider how your online presence impacts the trust that your patients and colleagues have in you. Never post anything that might violate this trust. This includes your "private" social media profiles. Often, a private post that was meant only for someone's friends and families get out into the public. Everything you post online – no matter where you post it – is a reflection of your personality, values, and priorities. If a patient or colleague sees you acting foolish at the bar, posing with weapons, or (gasp) sharing details of a surgery or patient, the ramifications can cause lasting damage on your career and practice.

Amazing Role Models

I've found that the best way to learn is to see examples of other physicians rocking the social media world. In this section, I'll list physicians, healthcare professionals, and organizations who are hitting it out of the park with their social media presence.

These doctors and organizations have been successful in increasing awareness about their practice, sharing information to their patients about their healthcare specialty, and have positioned themselves as thought leaders in the field to colleagues.

Step by Step Pediatrics

Step by Step Pediatrics is a general pediatrician's office in Westerville, Ohio, with five resident MDs. They pride themselves on "comprehensive pediatric care from birth to adolescence."

Active On
Facebook, Twitter, YouTube, and LinkedIn

Target Audience
Step by Step Pediatrics considers educating their families a top priority. They are by far the most active on Facebook, where they educate parents about child nutrition, vaccinations, mental health information for children and teens, local epidemiology and disease, and common need-to-knows for parents. They also share updates about their practice so their patients know what's changing and what to expect.

Why Their Social Media Presence Is on Point
Step by Step Pediatrics uses their Facebook to educate and connect with parents. Although they're on multiple social media channels, their Facebook page is the best.

- They use Facebook to improve *transparency*. Patients can easily see what's going on in the office, who works there, and what they can expect from their visit. Through Facebook, they get a sense of the attitudes and personalities of the doctors and staff at Step by Step Pediatrics. A great way they achieve this is by sharing updates about their practice (such as the fact that they just started screening teenagers for depression and why it's such an important step.) They even share pictures of their lost and found pile to ask patients to claim what they lost.
- They also achieve transparency by putting their doctors and staff in front of the Facebook cameras. They introduce new team members and share the personal medical opinions of their doctors. Furthermore, they'll have one of their doctors post a video to educate patients. One video, of their own Dr. Miller, educates parents about what to keep in mind over the summer for child safety. This way, patients get to know the doctors before they even step into the office.
- They ***educate***! They share reputable articles about health, medicine, safety, nutrition, and wellness that's rooted in cutting-edge research and studies. They share information about parenting tips and ideologies, mental health issues in children and teens, how to ensure healthy eating patterns in kids, how to assist smooth childhood transitions (like starting the school year), and how to talk to kids about drugs and sexually transmitted infections (Fig. 7.2). Based on their engagement patterns, their parents remain engaged with Step by Step Pediatrics because they

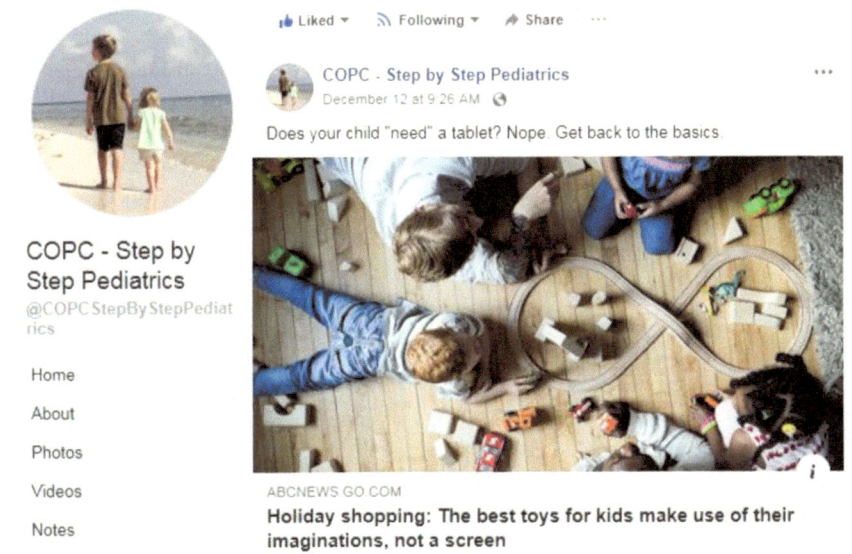

Does your child "need" a tablet? Nope. Get back to the basics.

ABCNEWS.GO.COM
Holiday shopping: The best toys for kids make use of their imaginations, not a screen

Fig. 7.2 Facebook page for a private practice. (Adapted from https://www.facebook.com/COPCStepByStepPediatrics/)

perceive the practice as being knowledgeable, and "up-to-date" on real-life concerns of modern parents.

- *Step by Step Pediatrics* is also not afraid to share slightly controversial information that's backed by medical science. They share this information with an unapologetic and passionate tone. For example, they shared an article from the Atlantic titled "Exercise Is ADHD Medication." They added a caption that said, "And anxiety medication. And depression medication. And overweight/obesity medication. And just what our kids should be doing every single day. The weather is finally nice. Send your kids outside to play."
- They connect with their patients through *humor*. They get that parenthood is hard. They know that parents will perceive the practice as more trustworthy if they show that they understand the challenges of parents in a way that makes them laugh. The use of tasteful humor also shows parents that the doctors at Step by Step Pediatrics "get it" and that they're real humans behind the white coat and framed diploma.
- All of their posts are *visual* and engaging. According to Kissmetrics [33], posts with photos on Facebook get 53% more likes, 104% more comments, and 84% more clicks on links than text-only posts. Photo posts account for 93% of the most engaging posts on Facebook and receive 39% more interaction overall.
- They *respond* to comments to further foster a sense of community, to answer questions, and to dispel confusion and myths.
- Their online voice is *competent*, *informative*, and *nonjudgmental* with a hint of being playful.

How They Curate Content

Step By Step Pediatrics provides a mix of content. Sometimes they'll create their own content by uploading their own videos and images from inside their practice. But most of the time, their content is curated from other places, such as articles from major publications and outlets, and even humorous articles from Huffington Post when they want to share a good laugh. They'll also share funny memes to connect with parents. Their favorite content to share is well-written, in-depth articles from major news outlets and publications about child health, nutrition, safety, and well-being from infancy into the teen years.

Wendy Sue Swanson MD

Wendy Sue Swanson MD is a pediatrician in Seattle Washington. She is best known for her blog titled Seattle Mama Doc, which aims to educate mothers (and all parents) about how to keep kids safe and healthy. She runs a podcast as well, which spans topics that range from infant car seats to drowning prevention to the importance of play for kids. From her biography on the Seattle Children's Hospital Website [34], she says, "I am passionate about improving the way media discusses pediatric health news and influences parents' decisions when caring for their children."

Active on
Facebook, Twitter.

Target Audience
Parents, specifically new and expecting moms. Sometimes, her posts are aimed toward fellow providers.

Why Her Social Media Presence Is on Point
- Online, Dr. Swanson's *general tone* makes it clear that she understands what parents are going through. When she speaks, it's clear that she's a pediatrician who is also a parent. This garners trust and a sense of rapport in her audience.
- She informs parents about *highly relevant health and safety information*: she shares information about gun safety, food allergies, social media use in teens, anxiety in new mothers, child nutrition, and more.
- She positions herself as the expert by *sharing her professional opinion* often. She shares much of her own, original content which adds validity. To read more about how healthcare professionals can create their own social media content (and why they should); refer to Chap. 8!
- Although Dr. Swanson is a pediatrician, she addresses the health concerns of the parents as well. With an understanding that parent health has a direct impact on the health of children, she dives into mental and physical health concerns of parents, specifically mothers. Whether reminding parents to spend less time on their smartphones or discussing with new moms how to lower their anxiety, Dr. Swanson is always looking out for the health of moms, too.

- She doesn't just leave a news story for parents to scroll past. Whenever she shares news stories (such as dangerous teen fads), she discusses with parents on how to address these issues with their kids. She doesn't just share content; she explains why she's sharing it, why it's relevant, and how people can take action in their own lives.

How She Curates Content

Dr. Swanson frequently *creates* a lot of her own content through podcasts, blogs, and videos. (See Chap. 8, about how and why to create your own content for social media.) But when she *curates* content, she shares external sources thoughtfully. She often shares articles from sources she trusts that share science-backed studies and research (Fig. 7.3).

Dr. Swanson also acts as an advocate when there's any major change in medical understanding, requirements, or news. For example, when the American Academy of Pediatrics changed their guidelines for child car seats, she shared the new guidelines and "broke them down" in terms that parents could more easily understand.

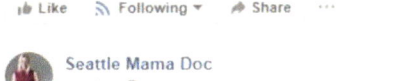

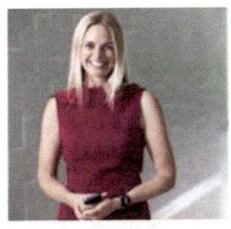

Seattle Mama Doc
@SeattleMamaDoc

Home

About

Posts

SoundCloud

Videos

Photos

Content Capsule

Community

Info and Ads

Seattle Mama Doc
July 31

The American Academy of Pediatrics recently published a new policy statement warning parents about food additives and chemicals children consume in food. There's no question that babies and children may be more vulnerable to the effects of toxins in our food source as their bodies, organs, and minds form.

Don't freak out - we can't control everything - but do decrease your use of plastics as much as you can. Here are some additional steps you can take to reduce risk and exposures from an interview I did with Today Show.

#BPAs #Phthalates #healthyeating #organic #foodsafety

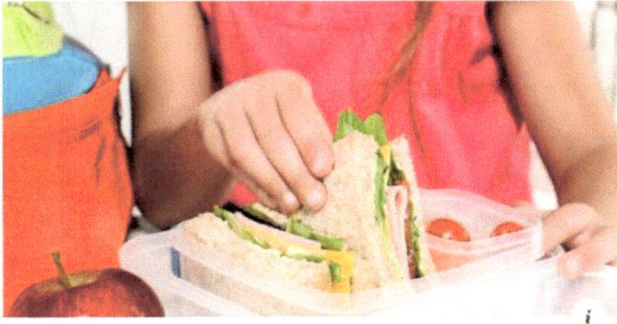

TODAY.COM
Pediatricians sound alarm about food additives and children's health

Fig. 7.3 Example of a Facebook page from a physician who shares evidence-based information. (Adapted from https://www.facebook.com/SeattleMamaDoc/)

She has a knack for attaching her "why" and her opinion so that parents can understand the context of the information she shares.

Dr. Kevin Pho

Dr. Kevin Pho is a physician of internal medicine who practices in New Hampshire. He spent a couple of years working as a physician researcher for Google Answers and realized that patients were not getting the information they needed in the examination room. Thus, he began his blog, KevinMD, where he and many other healthcare professionals discuss the realities of the American healthcare system and the everyday challenges that doctors face. Dr. Pho is often invited to be a keynote speaker, probably due to his prolific social media presence. He is also on the *USA Today* board of contributors, where he runs a commentary on doctor welfare and the American healthcare system.

Active on
Twitter

Target Audience
Healthcare professionals

Why His Social Media Presence Is on Point
- Dr. Pho's social media presence is a light in the dark for physicians who need a place that understands what doctor's face on a daily basis. On his Twitter page, he exclusively shares articles from his blog that discusses doctor burnout, difficult patient decisions, and how doctors can practice self-care and stay vigilant about their mental health.
- He frequently shares articles written by other doctors and healthcare professionals, which means that his Twitter feed introduces multiple voices from across the medical landscape. This offers different perspectives and dynamic conversations.
- His social media flow is highly consistent. He tends to focus on the same topics within the healthcare professional realm: the pay gap, alternatives to prescribing opioids, mental health in the medical field, doctor burnout, and medical school debt.
- Dr. Pho is a great example of social media syndication. By sharing his blog articles on Twitter (Fig. 7.4), he channels traffic to his website and back to Twitter from his blog. Everything is connected.

How He Curates Content
It is rare that Dr. Pho writes anything of his own. In fact, on the "About" page on KevinMD, it says, "Thousands of authors contribute to KevinMD.com [35]: frontline primary care doctors, surgeons, specialist physicians, nurses, medical students, policy experts. And of course, patients, who need the medical profession to hear

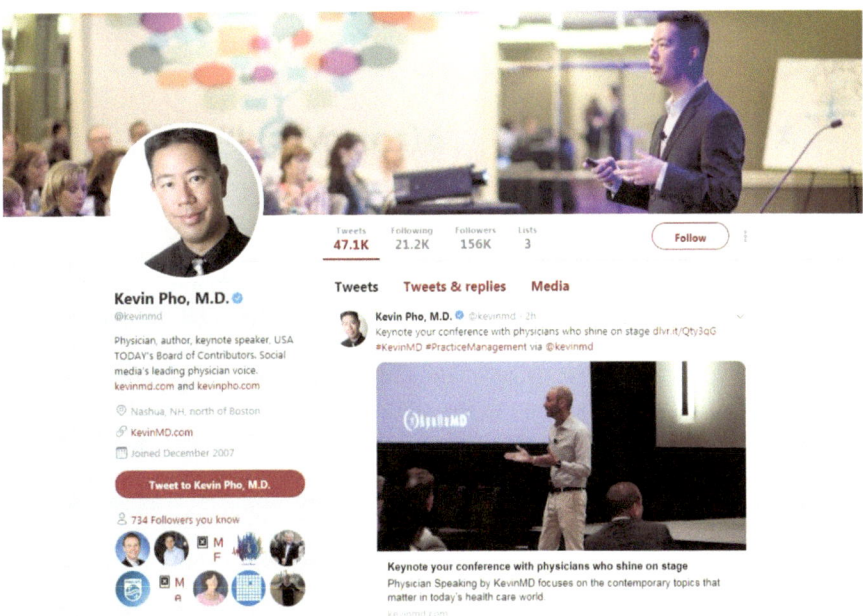

Fig. 7.4 Twitter page for Kevin Pho, MD, creator of the popular KevinMD website. (Adapted from https://twitter.com/kevinmd)

their voices." This makes for a diverse content base that allows readers to see issues from all sides.

Instead of creating his own content, Kevin allows a space for many other physicians to share their own ideas and concerns in a supportive environment meant for the personal and professional growth of healthcare professionals.

Dr. Dave Stukus @AllergyKidsDoc

Dr. Dave Stukus is a pediatric allergy and asthma specialist at Nationwide Children's Hospital in Columbus, Ohio, where he serves as the Director of the hospital's Complex Asthma Clinic. He's a top Twitter influencer in the country, with 16 thousand followers, and growing. (He also wrote a couple of chapters in this book!) According to his Twitter profile, he's "dispelling myths one tweet at a time," and he does so with humor and ample research to back him up.

Dr. Stukus tells me that his career really started taking off once he became really involved on Twitter and garnered a loyal following. Because of his strong and consistent Twitter presence, Dr. Stukus has been invited to give speeches and lectures by organizations looking to hear his outlook. More patients seek him out because his info-sharing on social media leads to higher perceived trust and a higher expectation for the medical care experience. Stukus is a perfect example of how showing your passion online can help people see how passionate you *are*!

Active on
Twitter

Target Audience
Families of children with asthma and food allergies. Anyone who wants to know more about medicine and diagnostics from a doctor's perspective

Why His Social Media Presence Is on Point
- Stukus has mastered a consistent voice of authority and humor. He understands how to be credible while also making his audience laugh. He frequently shares information about asthma and allergies in a funny yet informative manner.
- Stukus' strategy is very consistent. He stays on the course of dispelling pervasive health myths, while backing up his claims with research, and often sharing a punchy gif to add a flare of personality.
- He points out articles that spread false information and raises awareness about the prevalence of false health information online.

How He Curates Content
Dr. Stukus is big on sharing articles from both sides of the credibility aisle, pointing out who to trust and who not to trust. He busts prevalent health myths with mirth and humor, sharing infographics, charts, and GIFs that educate on how to identify faulty health claims online. But he doesn't just share the false info – he often shares articles and studies that he deems important and relevant.

Otherwise, Dr. Stukus creates his own content here and there, whether it's a quick video to share what he's thinking, an announcement about an upcoming event he's attending or speech he's giving, and of course, the occasional corny joke.

Dr. Eric Topol

Dr. Topol is an excellent example of how smart social media use can help position physicians as thought leaders. Not that he needed much help in this department. Dr. Topol has received international acclaim for his groundbreaking research in individualized medicine [36]. He has spent his career researching the clinical development of new drugs and devices and has also researched the interplay of genomics and medicine. Specializing in cardiovascular disease and internal medicine, Dr. Topol's Twitter feed has become a major news source for his followers, spanning topics from nutrition to cardiovascular health, to cancer, and to medical technology and beyond.

Active on
Twitter

Target Audience
Physicians and scientists

Why His Social Media Presence Is on Point

Dr. Topol's Twitter feed reflects what he stands for as a physician, scientist, and researcher. He challenges medical dogma by sharing groundbreaking studies that question the medical status quo. He's a go-to for cutting-edge medical findings, and he has a good commentary on the healthcare system and how physicians can work toward better human health outcomes.

- He curates recent medical findings and breakthroughs (big and small) and acts as a center-of-the-wheel for medical news that physicians would have to spend hours trying to find.
- He shares articles and studies while highlighting the most essential passages, for a quick read-through.
- He comments on how to cut through misconceptions and long-held beliefs in the face of new research and data.
- He shakes things up a bit by sharing comics and easy-read consumer articles that touch on genomics, the healthcare industry, and medical technology.
- He isn't afraid of taking a stance on politically charged topics, which helps readers see his honesty.

How He Curates Content

Dr. Topol keeps tabs on the latest medical breakthroughs and news, so he can syndicate it to his followers. He shares medical studies and consumer articles that any healthcare professional would find relevant and interesting, and he makes it easy for readers to "get the gist," by providing commentary and highlighting essential passages.

In the midst of heavy, hard-hitting research, he lightens things up a bit by sharing relevant comics about the current state of medical technology, healthcare, and the like. He's focused very much on being a news source and thought leader for physicians, scientists, and researchers, so he pulls the best, most intriguing, groundbreaking findings and shares them for the world to see (Fig. 7.5).

Examples of Excellent Content

For the physician who doesn't know where to start when it comes to curating content on social media, I've come up with some ideas to get you started. As you get better and more fluent with social media, you'll find that you have your favorite go-to's for content curation. Maybe you'll be all about the inspirational quotes. Maybe you'll share helpful tips. Maybe you'll share groundbreaking studies or articles. Whatever you choose, it mostly matters to just stay consistent and to share the highest-quality content you can find. So here are some ideas to get you started (or to get you going!). And know that you'll find the content that's right for you.

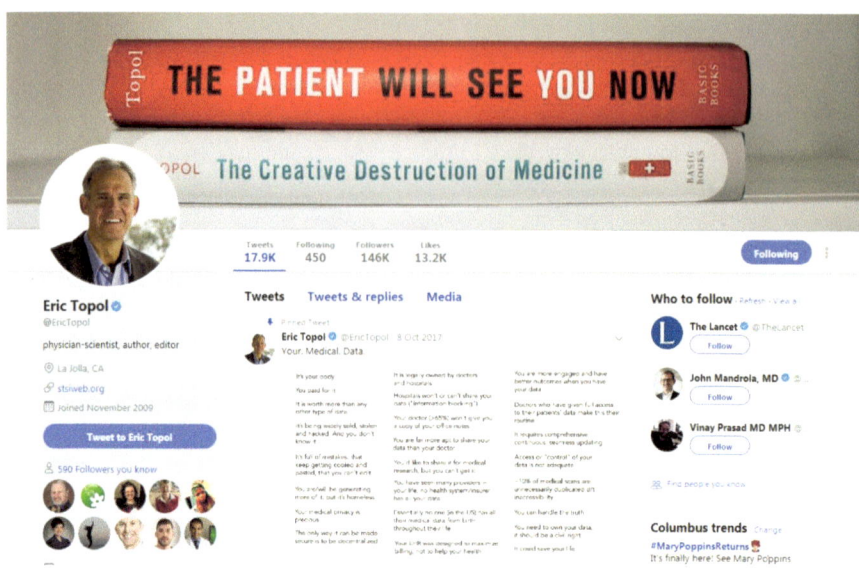

Fig. 7.5 Twitter page for Eric Topol, MD. (Adapted from https://twitter.com/EricTopol)

Amazing Content Ideas

• Latest news and emerging trends.

Pro tip: Google Alerts is a wonderful source for staying up to date on the latest news. Their tagline says it all: "Monitor the web for interesting new content."

Twitter trending is another great resource if you want to explore the most popular, buzzing topics that are currently being discussed more than others on the platform.

• Share helpful tips.

As a specialist, researcher, scientist, or healthcare professional, you probably have some health tips and tricks up your sleeve that your followers never even think about.

• Share content by other experts in your field.

This is a great way to start relationships and to engage your audience. Besides, people love it when you share their content on Twitter. It's a great way to make a new follower (and fan)!

- Share visuals!

Photos, GIFs, infographics, and videos are a great way to increase reader engagement. I've seen medical practices use video and photos to share behind-the-scenes info about their practice, and I've seen doctors use infographics to get a point across. I've also seen doctors use GIFs with abandonment in order to connect with readers through humor and expression.

- Quotes from experts in your field.

You probably have role models in your field that you've looked up to for a while. Maybe you read their books, follow them on social, and have been inspired by their thoughts and actions. Leverage what inspires you. It will probably inspire someone else, too.

- Don't shy from your own opinions.

When doctors take a stance on how to improve health outcomes and how to improve the healthcare industry, it shows patients that the doctors are informed, engaged, and genuinely care about public health. Add your own thoughtful commentary to the issue and hone your own voice as a professional.

- Draw from studies to create your own posts.

Chances are, you're one of the few people who can break down the newest studies to your patients. Serve up some valuable, cutting-edge health information by elucidating the major takeaways from new studies for lay audiences.

- Curate screenshots to illustrate content.

Visual elements will always help you reach higher engagement, especially for complex topics. If you see something you'd love to share on social media, make sure you carry over any visual content so the material carries more impact.

- Generate conversations by asking questions or sharing something semi-controversial.

Again, there's no reason to fear the validity of your own opinions when it comes to topics that are semi-controversial or political. If you know something's right, it's perfectly okay to share. Asking your audience questions is another great way to get a conversation going and is also useful in better understanding your audience.

- Share preventative healthcare content.

Whatever your specialty is, chances are, you could be educating your readers on how to avoid a certain undesirable outcome. Avoid skin cancer by slathering on sunscreen! Avoid Alzheimer's disease by getting enough exercise! Avoid diabetes by cutting sugar intake! Especially if your audience is comprised of patients, this type of info is always a big hit.

- Raise awareness for your favorite campaigns and programs.

Is there a cause you care deeply about? Is there a program your hospital is running that you think is a major win? Use social media to share it!

- Raise awareness about local health issues.

Oftentimes, health issues vary by location. Is air pollution extra bad in the valley where you live, affecting asthma patients? Are there algae blooms that make it a health hazard to swim at the lakeshore? Sometimes, your patients will need more information about a health condition because they live near the risk.

- Build awareness between practitioners in your field.

This is a big one, especially if your prime audience is other healthcare professionals. Share the studies; share the articles. Be a knowledge source for others in your specialty. It can get a great conversation going that can get great minds thinking.

Conclusion

More and more doctors are logging onto social media and pulling their favorite articles, studies, images, infographics, and more from around the web. They're sharing health information with their patients, groundbreaking studies with their peers, and creating more awareness for their practices. If more and more physicians and healthcare professionals curate content online, they can change the online conversation around health for the better and propel their careers into the next level.

References

1. Company info. Facebook Newsroom, Facebook 2018, https://newsroom.fb.com/company-info/.
2. Balakrishnan A, Boorstin J. Instagram says it now has 800 million users, up 100 million since April. CNBC, 25 Sept 2017, www.cnbc.com/2017/09/25/how-many-users-does-instagram-have-now-800-million.html.
3. Twitter: number of active users 2010–2018. Statista, 2018, www.statista.com/statistics/282087/number-of-monthly-active-twitter-users/.
4. Von Muhlen M, Ohno-Machado L. Reviewing social media use by clinicians. PubMed.gov, U.S. National Library of Medicine, Sept 2012, www.ncbi.nlm.nih.gov/pubmed/22759618/.
5. U.S. population with a social media profile 2018. Statista, www.statista.com/statistics/273476/percentage-of-us-population-with-a-social-network-profile/.
6. Ventola CL. Social media and health care professionals: benefits, risks, and best practices. U.S. National Library of Medicine, July 2014, www.ncbi.nlm.nih.gov/pmc/articles/PMC4103576/.
7. Househ M. The use of social media in healthcare: organizational, clinical, and patient perspectives. PubMed.gov, U.S. National Library of Medicine, www.ncbi.nlm.nih.gov/pubmed/23388291/.

8. Lawhon L. New survey reveals importance of online health communities. Health Union, LLC, 15 June 2016, https://health-union.com/news/online-health-experience-survey/.

9. Shearer EI, Gottfried J. News use across social media platforms 2017. Pew Research Center's Journalism Project, 7 Sept 2017, www.journalism.org/2017/09/07/news-use-across-social-media-platforms-2017/.

10. Duggan M, et al. Parents and social media I Pew Research Center. Pew Research Center: Internet, Science & Tech, 22 May 2017, www.pewinternet.org/2015/07/16/parents-and-social-media/.

11. Migala J. 3 things to know about medical advice on social media. Parents, www.parents.com/parenting/better-parenting/advice/3-things-to-know-about-medical-advice-on-social-media/.

12. Fox S, Purcell K. Social media and health I Pew Research Center. Pew Research Center: Internet, Science & Tech, 3 Jan 2014, www.pewinternet.org/2010/03/24/social-media-and-health/.

13. Fowler FJ, et al. Informing and involving patients to improve the quality of medical decisions. Health Affairs, Apr 2011, www.healthaffairs.org/doi/full/10.1377/hlthaff.2011.0003.

14. Metzger MJ, Flanagin AJ. Using Web 2.0 technologies to enhance evidence-based medical information. Curr Neurol Neurosci Rep, U.S. National Library of Medicine, www.ncbi.nlm.nih.gov/pubmed/21843095/.

15. Grindrod K, et al. Pharmacy 2.0: a scoping review of social media use in pharmacy. Curr Neurol Neurosci Rep, U.S. National Library of Medicine, www.ncbi.nlm.nih.gov/pubmed/23810653/.

16. Westerman D, et al. Social media as information source: recency of updates and credibility of information. The Canadian Journal of Chemical Engineering, Wiley-Blackwell, 8 Nov 2013., https://onlinelibrary.wiley.com/doi/full/10.1111/jcc4.12041.

17. Gray R. Future - lies, propaganda and fake news: a challenge for our age. BBC News, BBC, 1 Mar 2017, www.bbc.com/future/story/20170301-lies-propaganda-and-fake-news-a-grand-challenge-of-our-age.

18. Anderson J, Rainie L. The future of truth and misinformation online I pew research center. Pew Research Center: Internet, Science & Tech, Pew Research Center: Internet, Science & Tech, 25 Apr 2018, www.pewinternet.org/2017/10/19/the-future-of-truth-and-misinformation-online/.

19. Vogel L. Viral misinformation threatens public health. Curr Neurol Neurosci Rep, U.S. National Library of Medicine, 18 Dec 2017, www.ncbi.nlm.nih.gov/pmc/articles/PMC5738254/.

20. Thon FM, Jucks R. Believing in expertise: how authors' credentials and language use influence the credibility of online health information. Health Commun J. 2017;32:828–36. www.tandfonline.com/doi/abs/10.1080/10410236.2016.1172296?src=recsys&journalCode=hhth20

21. Hou J, Shim M. The role of provider-patient communication and trust in online sources in Internet use for health-related activities. Curr Neurol Neurosci Rep, U.S. National Library of Medicine, www.ncbi.nlm.nih.gov/pubmed/21154093.

22. Health information-seeking behavior of seniors who use the Internet: a survey. J Med Internet Res, JMIR Publications Inc., Toronto, Canada, www.jmir.org/2015/1/e10/.

23. Evaluating health information. UCSF Medical Center, www.ucsfhealth.org/education/evaluating_health_information/.

24. Joyce M. Conflicts of interest in medicine: pervasive, worrisome, and detrimental to healthcare. HealthNewsReview.org, 17 Jan 2017, www.healthnewsreview.org/2017/01/123967/.

25. Boachie P. Social media marketing statistics 2016 and beyond. Digitimatic, 4 Sept 2017., www.digitimatic.com/social-media-marketing-statistics/.

26. Peck JL. Social media in nursing education: responsible integration for meaningful use. Curr Neurol Neurosci Rep, U.S. National Library of Medicine, Mar 2014., www.ncbi.nlm.nih.gov/pubmed/24530130/.

27. Atheunis ML. Patients' and health professionals' use of social media in health care: motives, barriers and expectations. NeuroImage, Academic Press, 27 July 2013, www.sciencedirect.com/science/article/pii/S0738399113002656.

28. Sarasohn-Kahn J. The wisdom of patients: health care meets online social media. California Healthcare Foundation, Apr 2008, www.chcf.org/wp-content/uploads/2017/12/PDF-HealthCareSocialMedia.pdf.

29. Househ M. The use of social Media in Healthcare: organizational, clinical, and patient perspectives. Curr Neurol Neurosci Rep, U.S. National Library of Medicine, 2013., www.ncbi.nlm.nih.gov/pubmed/23388291/.
30. Farnan J, et al. Online medical professionalism: patient and public relationships: policy statement from the American College of Physicians and the Federation of State Medical Boards. Curr Neurol Neurosci Rep, U.S. National Library of Medicine, 16 Apr 2013., www.ncbi.nlm.nih.gov/pubmed/23579867/.
31. Blendon RJ, Benson JM. Public trust in physicians – U.S. medicine in international perspective I NEJM. N Engl J Med, Oct 2014, www.nejm.org/doi/full/10.1056/NEJMp1407373#t=article.
32. Thom DH, et al. Measuring patients' trust in physicians when assessing quality of care. Health Aff, 2014., www.healthaffairs.org/doi/full/10.1377/hlthaff.23.4.124.
33. Cooper BB. 7 powerful Facebook statistics you should know about. Fast Company, Fast Company, 12 Dec 2013, www.fastcompany.com/3022301/7-powerful-facebook-statistics-you-should-know-about.
34. Know more about Dr. Wendy sue Swanson. Seattle Mama Doc, seattlemamadoc.seattlechildrens.org/about-this-blog/.
35. Pho K, et al. Be heard on social media's leading physician voice. KevinMD.com, www.kevinmd.com/blog/heard-social-medias-leading-physician-voice.
36. Topol E. Scripps health, www.scripps.org/physicians/5497-eric-topol?tab=overview.

Content Creation

8

Kathryn E. Nuss

If you build it, they will come.

—Ray Kinsella, Field of Dreams

Building an Assortment of Unique Content

Not many physicians are creating their own content on social media. As of 2017, only about 1% of physicians were creating and publishing their own content on social media. In contrast, about 9% of physicians share non-original content. More still contribute to online discussions and forums. Most doctors are passive consumers on social media – using the Internet to find relevant medical information related to their patients, specialty, or practice. When we put this all together, we see that 80% of physicians are logging into social media, but only 1% of them are producing original content [1].

This seems like a missed opportunity when you take into account that nearly half of all patients are logging onto social media in order to find more information about a certain doctor or health professional. Patients are looking for their next doctor on social media, but what many of these patients find are bare social media pages or nothing at all. Maybe they'll find a business listing on Google Maps and a couple of pictures if they're lucky. It makes sense that doctors take advantage of this free and easy opportunity to land new patients and to instill trust and confidence in the process.

Whether you are a physician, a nurse practitioner, or a dietitian, your social media presence (or lack thereof) can make all the difference between your practices looking like a sleepy backwater versus looking like a cutting-edge facility.

This might be a huge reason why, after weighing the benefits and risks of social media content creation, more and more healthcare professionals are deciding to log on and connect.

© Springer Nature Switzerland AG 2019
D. R. Stukus et al., *Social Media for Medical Professionals*,
https://doi.org/10.1007/978-3-030-14439-5_8

Why Original Content?

Most professionals reading this will at least have their own personal Facebook page. Others will have a LinkedIn account they haven't updated in a while, a personal Instagram where they post pictures of sushi and yard work, and maybe they'll log into Pinterest when they feel inspired to look up mermaid party decor for their daughter's fourth birthday party.

But when it comes to having professional social media accounts, some healthcare professionals are reluctant to jump on the bandwagon. "After all," they think, "It's not like I run a restaurant. I'm not an entrepreneur. I'm not selling LuLaroe or trying to get people to hit up my Etsy shop. I'll just share some health articles on my professional Twitter and call it a day."

This is all well and good, but depending on your goals, there are significant advantages to creating your own content. First off, there's a lot of health information out there, but not much of it is doctor-generated content. Most of our patients are getting health information from yoga teachers, self-proclaimed crystal masters, 22-year-old freelance writers, and other people who have never been to medical school. Maybe their information is on point, and maybe it's not. Healthcare professionals creating original content means there's more accurate health information on the Internet. This helps your patients, and it helps your practice.

Creating your own content is also a chance to manage your reputation more effectively. There are healthcare practices that have no online presence, which means if any prospective patients want to learn more about them, they have to rely on patient reviews and random pictures they can find on google. It could be the best pediatrician in central Ohio, but if they have less-than-positive reviews, no website, and some blurry cellphone pictures of their building, prospective patients aren't going to get the best impression.

So yes, creating your own content is as much about education as it is about marketing. Think of it this way: social media helps to satisfy the needs of the patients while also satisfying the needs of the hospital, doctor, or medical practice. The patient needs accurate health information. They also need an informed doctor. The doctor needs patients. The practice needs people to consider them the best medical professionals for the job. Creating your own content allows you to construct that narrative, to educate about who you are as a healthcare professional, what your practice is about, and how you go about caring for patients.

The SEO Factor

If you ever go on the Internet, chances are that you've heard the term SEO in recent years. SEO stands for "Search Engine Optimization" and refers to bolstering a website's visibility in search rankings. The goal is to get on the first page of a google search. For example, when a patient types in "Chest Pain," an original video or blog on your website can pop up in search rankings, leading the patient to your digital doorstep. Even better, if a patient types "Pediatricians in Columbus Ohio specializing in Allergies," you can bet that your original content on your website is going to pull your website to the top of Google's list of relevant sites.

Marketers definitely know the ins and outs of good SEO. Of marketers polled, 72% found that creating original content was the most effective SEO tactic. Why? Because search engines like Google like seeing websites that are continuously and routinely updated with new content. That means writing new blog posts and uploading new videos. Content creation goes a long way in helping patients find your practice online.

According to Pew Research, 72% of internet users looked online for health information within the past year [2]. More than ever before, patients are jumping online to find health information. Creating original content ensures that these new patients can find you.

With this in mind, it's a good idea to focus on regional and local SEO. The Internet is a huge place, and it won't benefit you to attract patients that are on the other side of the planet. Instead, targeting your original content toward your local community will ensure that the people in your town can find you online.

When it comes to SEO, it's all about the keywords. Peppered throughout your content, make sure you have relevant words to the audience you're trying to attract. Is the audience comprised of men 50 years and older who suffer from prostate cancer in the greater Cincinnati area? If this is the case, you would include the words "prostate cancer" and "Cincinnati" in your content. This ensures that when a patient types their query into the Google search bar, your website pops up because it shares much of the same verbiage.

Sometimes You Have to Create Your Own Content

Creating your own content as a physician or healthcare professional is often considered a "nice-to-have." But sometimes there are situations where it's hard to *avoid* creating your own content. When you have to communicate something that's specific to your practice or specialty to your patients, then you really have to create the content yourself.

Administrative Organization and Social Media

Before social media took over, doctor's offices could really only communicate with their patients via phone or mail. In order to talk to the doctor, patients had to call and wait on the line. If there was an office closing, changed office hours, or scheduling changes, there was no real, central way to communicate this to patients. In order to do anything, patients had to pick up the phone. Our patients' days of being put on hold are now mercifully over.

When it comes to administrative tasks such as posting office hours, announcing closings, and communicating about appointment scheduling, there's no choice but to create your own content on social media. First of all, our patients are logged on already. We don't have to direct them to some other web address that's "out of their way." We're catching them where they already are and sharing information that's helpful to them and helps our practices run smoothly. (And it keeps the phone lines free!)

By creating our own content, we can also direct and inform patients on how we operate. We can show them how to easily book appointments, what our office hours are, where we're located, and what they need to bring (if anything) to appointments. Making it easy on our patients could be the difference between patients coming to us for services, instead of the doctor on the other side of town.

Local Health Concerns

It's necessary to create your own content when you live in an area with specific health concerns. Of course, the healthcare content produced in Hawaii is going to focus on different issues than healthcare content in Maine. Perhaps you live in an area with unique health concerns. Do you live in an area with higher-than-average air pollution? Are ticks especially bad in your area? Is there a whooping cough epidemic going around your city? Is there a general misunderstanding about the safety of vaccines in your neighborhood? These are all local issues that might have to be addressed by writing your own blog posts, filming your own videos, or even just creating your own visual Facebook and Twitter posts that target the affected audiences. After all, you're here to help out with the health concerns of your local area. Your social media presence can spotlight you as the local expert who can help.

Developing a Content Plan

Content creation is made easier by having a plan. Social media content creation is not about throwing everything at the wall and seeing what sticks (okay, it's a little bit like that.) But before you start throwing anything, there are certain objectives and goals to have in mind. Get clear on how it will benefit you (and your audience) to create your own content on social media. Here are some common goals for why physicians and other healthcare professionals join social media:

- To advertise the services of their medical practice
- To attract new patients
- To understand their patients better by engaging in conversations with them, asking them questions, and getting a glimpse into their personal lives (e.g., if your patient keeps posting pictures of themselves puffing on cigarettes, you'll know how to serve them better)
- To become a cutting-edge voice in your specialty
- To connect with other professionals in your specialty or field
- To become a relevant news source for other doctors and healthcare professionals

- To become an accurate and trustworthy fountain of knowledge for patients and families online.

Knowing your goals for logging on is the first step in good content creation.

Your Content Creation Depends on Who Your Audience Is

Your audience informs your content, your persona, and your voice. Are you talking to young medical school students? Parents of children with cancer? Women who are interested in cosmetic surgery? Other cardiologists?

For example, if you're targeting new mothers, you probably won't want to share complex research studies only recognizable to healthcare professionals. Instead, you'll want to share content that resonates with new moms: how to tell if a bowel movement is normal. How to troubleshoot tummy troubles. How to get enough sleep when there's a newborn in the house.

Marketers develop what they call "buyer personas" when they're creating their content strategies. This includes getting specific on who the target audience is. So specific, in fact, that they add an age, gender, occupation, marital status, location, income, education level, values, fears, pain points, and desires. This helps marketers in a couple ways. It helps them cultivate trust in their consumers, helps them understand consumer needs better, and helps them build an effective strategy around messaging and imagery. Developing buyer personas can be helpful for healthcare professionals as well. Creating personas can help you discern the values of your audience, where they are (are they all on Facebook and can't stand Twitter?) and how you can create content that resonates with their needs.

Creating a Content Calendar

A huge part of having a content plan is putting together a content calendar. A content calendar helps you stay consistent and on track. It helps you avoid gaps in communicating with your audience. It even helps marketers come up with original ideas that they wouldn't have thought of on the fly. And by having a plan, you can be assured that your content marketing is supporting your big-picture goals for being on social media in the first place.

Some healthcare professionals worry that logging onto social media is a waste of time. But if you have a solid content strategy, with a plan, you'll see a solid return on investment.

Only 32% of marketers on social media have a content marketing strategy with a calendar, and those marketers are 60% more likely to consider their content marketing efforts effective, compared to those without a plan. This means that larger gains are seen when we don't fly by the seat of our pants, in both medicine and marketing [3].

There are three major steps to take when creating your content strategy:

Determine your Topics
Make sure they support your greater plan. If you're a cardiologist, you're not going to want to post recipes for your favorite food! I suggest that you come up with three major themes to post about. For example, if your specialty is obstetrics and gynecology, perhaps your topic of discussion will focus on breast health, fertility, and pregnancy.

Decide on which Platforms you're Going to Create Content
Don't try and establish a presence on all social media sites – you don't want to spread yourself too thin. Choose a couple of sites and stick with those for now. As you grow and expand, you can think about adding more later once you get established online. For example, maybe you'll run a blog on your website and share posts to Facebook and twitter.

Fill in the Content Calendar
Lastly, fill in the calendar. This calendar can either be a spreadsheet or be in your traditional block-calendar form, Fig. 8.1. As long as you get an idea for what to post when, you now have a content calendar that can lead you on an effective, strategic content creation plan.

MONDAY (DATE)				
Time	Title	Copy	Link	Clicks
	TWITTER			
0:00				
2:00				
4:00				
6:00				
8:00				
10:00				
12:00				
14:00				
16:00				
18:00				
20:00				
22:00				
	FACEBOOK			
6:00				
10:00				
2:00				
	GOOGLE+			
8:00				
10:00				
2:00				
	LINKEDIN			
8:00				
12:00				
4:00				
	INSTAGRAM			
12:00				
18:00				
TUESDAY (DATE)				
Time	Title	Copy	Link	Clicks
	TWITTER			

Fig. 8.1 Example of how a calendar can be utilized to organize social media posts

Platforms for Excellent Content Creation

With so many platforms out there on which you can create top-notch content, it's really up to you to decide which one works best for you. You'll probably want (or already have) a website, but beyond that, the possibilities are endless. You can film your own videos, write your own blogs, record monthly podcasts, or focus on just breaking down studies for lay audiences to understand. Here are a few platforms that can help you reach the widest audience possible.

A Website!

If you run your own practice, chances are, you have a website. A website is essential because it acts as your central hub for all elements of your content. It is the original place where all your content is stored, from blog posts to videos to podcasts; your website should have it all. When readers see your content on social media sites or YouTube, the content should always lead them back to your website.

Your website is also the first place that prospective and veteran patients alike are going to go to find answers, from services offered to hours to more information about the doctors, Fig. 8.2.

If you don't already have a website, website creation platforms such as WordPress and Weebly are a great place to start. These platforms are easy to use and result in professional sites within only a few hours.

Blog Posts

Your blog posts will be hosted on your website, so it's technically the same platform.

Blog posts are a great way to educate your audience and show that you're a thought leader in your niche. Having a blog conveys a level of expertise and passion

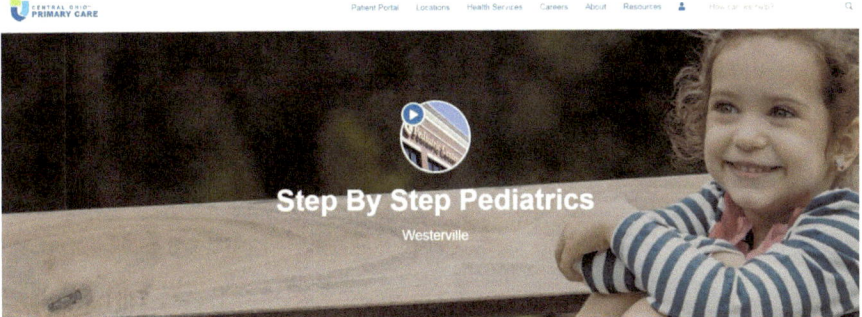

Fig. 8.2 Example of a website created by a private practice. (https://www.facebook.com/COPCStepByStepPediatrics/)

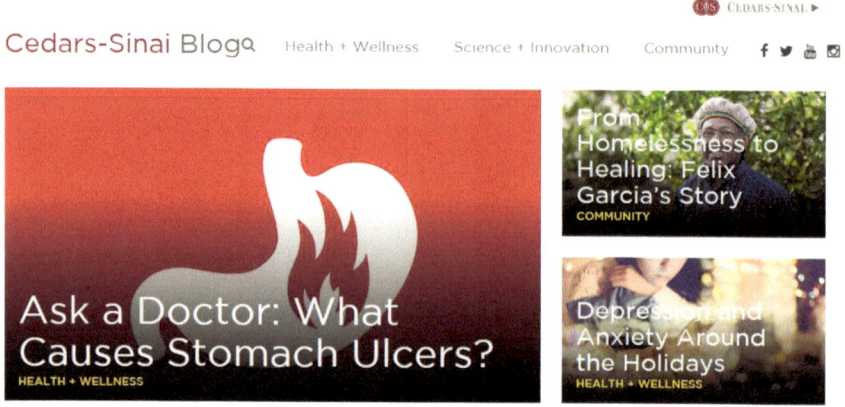

Fig. 8.3 Website created by a hospital system to share original blog posts. (https://blog.cedars-sinai.edu/)

in your specialty. It's the perfect way to educate patients, to dispel myths, and to reach a wide audience.

For inspiration, check out some physician blogs that deliver solid information to patients, and that make their organizations look like pros. Cedars-Sinai Blog goes beyond the goings-on at Cedars-Sinai and dives into topics that are interesting to everyone – from the science behind hangovers to knowing whether you really have food poisoning, to knowing the signs of human trafficking (Fig. 8.3). They cover it all, so it's easy to get sucked in and spend more time than intended on their blog!

Another great blog is the Dr. Leslie Greenberg blog. Dr. Greenberg runs her blog on WordPress and discusses topics that she feels are most useful for her patients and the rest of the world. She covers topics such as marijuana's effect on the adolescent brain, vaccines, women's health, and more.

When blogging, aesthetics matter, so take your time. Spend some time making sure the blog's design is how you want it to look. And speaking of SEO, there are right and wrong ways to write a blog post when it comes to optimizing search engine traffic to your website. Here's how to write for SEO:

- Use a headline with large font to highlight the main idea.
- Use subheadings to break apart ideas within the text and to keep scanners engaged.
- Write like a reporter! This means using the inverted pyramid structure. The beginning of the blog post should have the most important information, for less important points to follow. The least important information should be at the very end. This ensures that readers get the main point quickly.
- Break up the text with bullet points!

- There's an art and a science to good headlines. Make sure you're writing compelling headlines that attract attention, but don't make them too click-batey. Eighty percent of people read headlines, but only 20% read the entire article [4].

Facebook

For medical practices and hospitals, Facebook seems to be a necessity if you want to attract new patients. Every day, billions of people log onto Facebook, looking for health information, new healthcare providers, and trying to find answers about health conditions for themselves or their loved ones.

Facebook is perfect for getting the conversation started. Most doctors are already well-versed in how to navigate Facebook, and it's a great way to attract patients – as Facebook boasts the highest amount of members of all social media sites.

If you're an independent physician and not a hospital or medical practice, I would still suggest creating a "page" on Facebook instead of using your own personal profile. Dr. Kevin Pho's Facebook page is a perfect example of what I'm talking about, Fig. 8.4. He keeps everything professional, sharing stories from his blog. Everyone can like and follow his page.

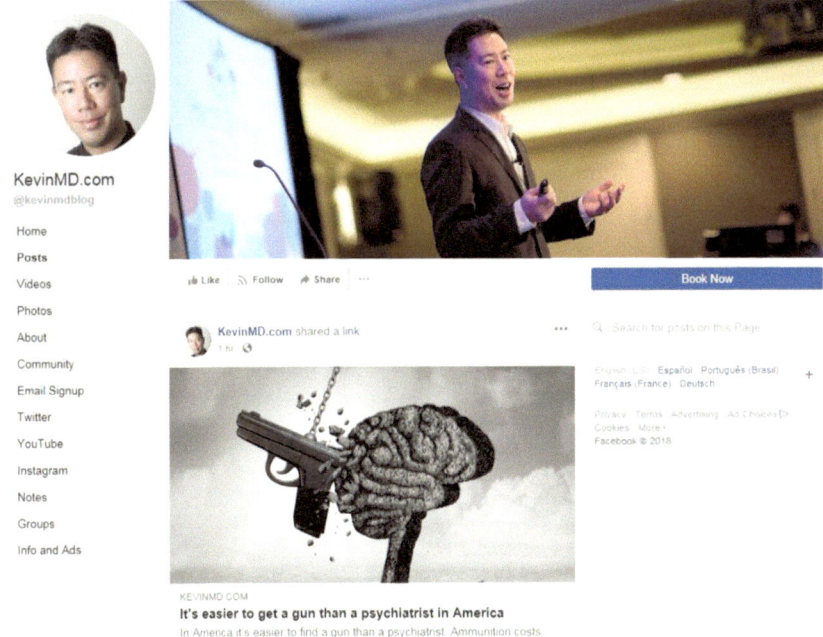

Fig. 8.4 Facebook page for Kevin Pho, MD. (https://www.facebook.com/kevinmdblog/)

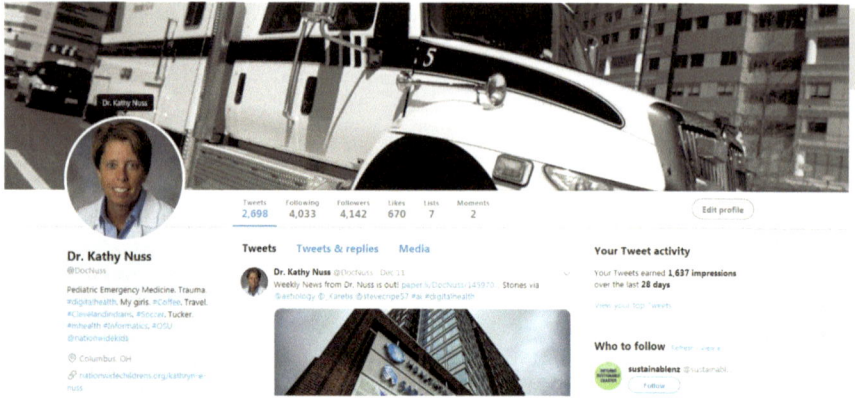

Fig. 8.5 Example of a healthcare professional using Twitter to connect with their target audience. (https://twitter.com/DocNuss)

Twitter

Twitter is perfect for professionals who want to connect with other professionals in their field, Fig. 8.5. With the use of hashtags, professionals in the same niche can connect on topics that interest them, from new studies and findings to how to handle certain patient scenarios. Twitter is a place where healthcare professionals can find their people, but it's less effective for hospitals and practices who want to attract new patients.

Twitter is great because it encourages the sharing of other people's posts, called "retweeting." The short-form content keeps everything short and sweet, which means it's great for those who aren't super confident in their writing skills.

LinkedIn

LinkedIn is perfect for physicians who are catering toward a professional audience of other healthcare professionals. You won't find much in the way of patients, but for the professional who is trying to reach students and other specialists in the field, LinkedIn is a great choice.

YouTube

YouTube is quickly rising in popularity among healthcare professionals who want to address frequently asked patient questions and to explain common procedures. Filming short videos allows hospitals, practices, and other healthcare facilities to show off their state-of-the-art facilities to would-be patients. It allows patients to see the provider in action and to get a sense for who she is before they even step into her office. Doctors can educate patients about their services and engage followers. Some doctors have even used short videos to show patients what to expect from a procedure and to allay anxieties.

Eric Strong, MD, runs a YouTube channel called "Strong Medicine: Free, On-demand videos for medical trainees and professionals" [5]. He has just over 215,000 subscribers, and he educates on topics that range from surviving medical school to how to interpret an X-ray, tips for new doctors, cardiology, and much more. He would love to see more doctors on YouTube, citing "Plenty of us are on Twitter, and there are plenty of physician blogs out there, but it feels like there are relatively few of us who avidly post on YouTube. And I don't understand why that's the case, because this is a wonderful platform for delivering free, open access medical education."

For filming video, it's always a good idea to invest in a high-quality camera. Ensure that both the lighting and the audio are excellent. You want to put your most professional foot forward!

Why Video Is King of the Social Media World

If you're trying to make an impact and stand out from the social media crowd, video is a surefire way to go. Here's why:

- Eighty-two percent of Twitter users watch video on the platform [6].
- Forty-five percent of people watch more than an hour of Facebook or YouTube videos a week. People prefer to watch a 30-second video than read a 5–7 paragraph blog post.
- Ninety-two percent of the time, viewers watching videos on a mobile device share the video with others [7].
- Video on social media generates 1200% more shares than text and images combined [8].

Podcast Platforms

If you feel that you have a face or comfort level better suited for radio, starting your own podcast can be a fun way to rap on relevant and important issues, in a way that doesn't rely on the more time-intensive video and blog routes. You don't have to write, and you don't have to edit video – you just have to know how to clearly talk about topics of interest.

Many podcasts are for doctors, by doctors, but some are meant to reach out to the patients themselves and, in some cases, parents of patients. Here in my hometown of Columbus Ohio, Dr. Mike Patrick runs a podcast called "PediaCast," associated with Nationwide Children's Hospital. PediaCast seeks to answer parent questions with the latest peer-reviewed journals and evidence-based answers, Fig. 8.6. He covers topics such as Baby hearing loss, West Nile Virus, Back to School, and much more [9].

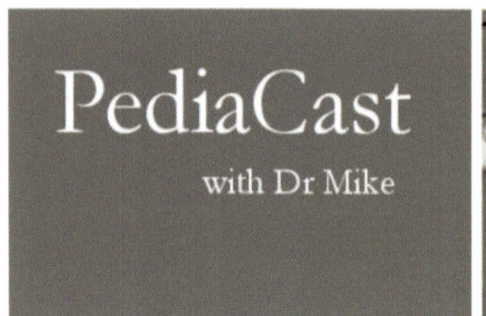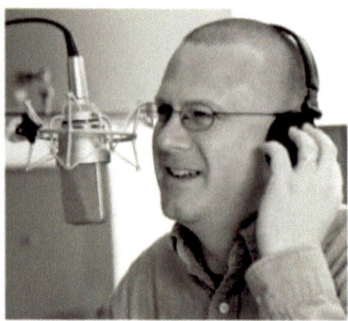

Welcome to PediaCast

A Pediatric Podcast for Parents

Fig. 8.6 Website for the popular PediaCast podcast. (https://www.pediacast.org/)

If making a podcast sounds exciting to you, there's a few different podcast platforms that are user-friendly, which include Libsyn, Podbean, Buzzsprout, SoundCloud, and others. You can share your podcast episodes on your website (much like you would a blog!), and when you publish new podcasts, you can share them over iTunes, Facebook, Twitter, and LinkedIn.

Instagram

Instagram is a highly visual platform that relies on a good aesthetic. The entirety of Instagram revolves around pictures that include short captions. Like Twitter, Instagram uses hashtags to connect people in similar niches and specialties.

Instagram is a great way for viewers to get a glimpse of the day-to-day life of a doctor, hospital, or medical practice. Dr. Michael Apa, a "dental rockstar," shares behind-the-scenes images and footage of his practice, and he frequently shares before-and-after photos of dental work to show off his expertise.

Another excellent use of Instagram in the medical field is by the Kaiser Family Foundation. They primarily share infographics about healthcare information in America. The Kaiser Family Foundation performs huge studies and writes papers, and their best findings make their way to Instagram.

Examples of Good Content Creation

You have a content strategy, a content calendar, and your platforms chosen. Now it's time to create some content! It can feel overwhelming starting from scratch – you have four followers – including your husband, sister, and mom, but not to worry! With the right content creation strategy, you'll be brimming with followers in no time. Here are some ideas to get you started.

Pull Together Studies as Quick Posts

It's always a good idea to elucidate the "gist" of the study in a couple of sentences, so your audience can immediately understand the conclusion of the study. Link to the study, so the people who want to dive in can!

Protip: Sign up for Google Alerts to get brand new alerts to your inbox on the newest material written about any topic. Looking for new info about heart health? Sodium intake? Diabetes? Sign up for Google Alerts so you have the newest info right in your inbox.

Curate Screenshots to Illustrate Content

When you're surfing the web, keep an eye out for compelling imagery that perfectly illustrates a factoid. For example, on Dr. David Stukus' Twitter, he shared a compelling diagram of how thunderstorms can exacerbate symptoms of asthma. Visuals are a compelling way to communicate content easily and effectively.

Pull Together the Latest News

Stay on top of the latest health news that appeals to your niche, and share it with a short sentence or two on your main takeaways. Health news and related topics can go a long way in educating your audience on the latest findings and research. But react fast! Share breaking news, experiences, and exchanges that are fresh and recent to engage your audience.

Curate Content Published by Top Sites in Your Niche

We all have our favorite health-related websites and blogs that we can't seem to get enough of. Even the best content creators pull from the top websites to support their points. Sometimes, nobody can say it better than that one other publication.

Post Powerful Quotes

If something inspires you, chances are, it'll inspire someone else. Cheer on those young med school students, help new parents relax a bit, and galvanize people to start eating right, all with some inspirational quotes.

Make Your Own GIFs or Share Your Favorite GIFs

GIFs are a great way to reference pop culture and make people laugh while pulling them into your content. Running the risk of boring content? Need to spice something up? Add a GIF. It'll make something funny and relatable in seconds, thereby spiking engagement.

Reference the Pamphlets from Your Own Office

Those pamphlets in your doctor's office are a great starting point for coming up with content. There might even be 3–4 social posts in 1 pamphlet! Be sure to include eye-catching imagery and clean, bright copy.

Record a Quick Video Educating About a Common Health Concern, Frequently Asked Health Questions, etc.

Videos get the best engagement on social media, and if you have a good camera, there's no reason you can't record a high-quality video in a matter of minutes!

Patient Testimonials

Testimonials are a powerful tool in attracting new patients. It boosts trust, and it's a great way to show gratitude to your patients! As discussed in depth in Chap. 9, patient privacy must always be accounted for when posting on social media. There are standard releases that patients can sign, allowing a medical practice or site to use their likeness or testimonial.

Podcasts

More and more people are listening to podcasts on their commutes, during workouts, and while making dinner. In fact, some people would rather listen to information than read it in blog form. If you're not a huge fan of writing or getting in front of a camera, this one's for you.

Fig. 8.7 Example of using infographics to discuss medical information. (https://www.cdc.gov/globalhealth/healthprotection/ghs/ghs-infographics.html)

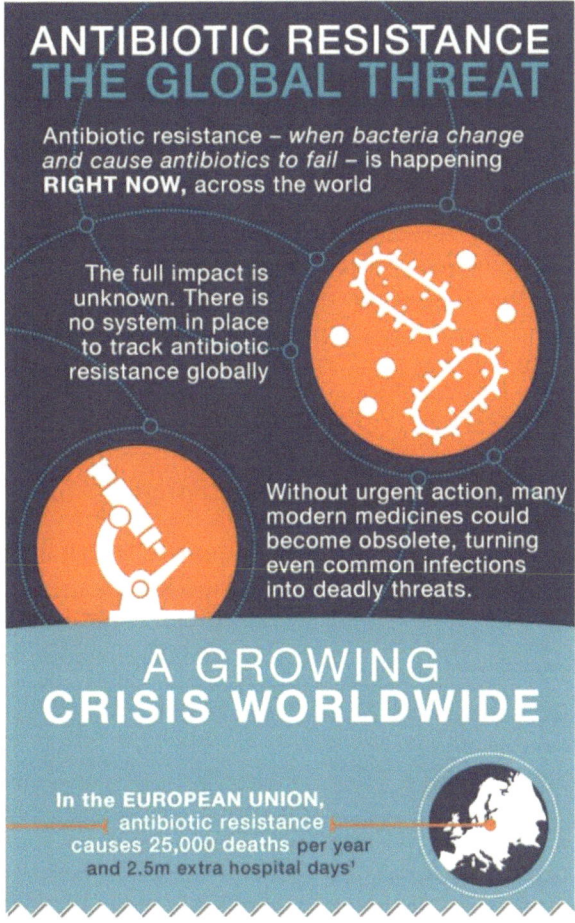

Create your Own Infographics

Tools such as Canva and Typorama make it easy to create your own infographics. If you have some tidbits of information you want to convey in a beautiful, visual way, then infographics are a surefire way to get reader's attention. Infographics are great because they're also highly likely to be shared, Fig. 8.7.

Exploit Trendy Topics

On Twitter's mobile apps, you can discover what's trending on the social media platform. Google Trends helps you identify what people are talking about online. Facebook has a "trending" section that helps you see what's popular today.

BuzzSumo helps you find the topics and content that performs best for any specialty or niche.

Organize Contests

This is an especially cute idea for doctor's offices and hospitals. It's a great way to rally the community around a particular topic. Ask for patient stories or rally cancer survivors around a hashtag that encourages patients to ask questions.

One particularly strong contest was done by UnitedHealthcare in their #WeDareYou Campaign. They encouraged followers to make one small positive health change in their lives per month and document it on social media. This helped them cultivate an online community of loyal and engaged followers.

Use High-Quality Stock Photography

Never forget that a visually pleasing post will always do better than a post with no imagery or poor imagery. Use high-quality pictures. If you don't have your own, don't be afraid to use high-quality stock photos from Canva, Pixabay, Stokpic, or Unsplash.

Cross-Promoting on Social Media

Say you have a website, a blog, and pages on Twitter, Facebook, and LinkedIn. When you write a blog post, you'll want to share that post on all your social platforms so that you can reach as many people as you possibly can. You'll want to tailor your message for each specific channel, making small tweaks to the content, imagery, and messaging, and to focus on the strengths and characteristics of each social platform.

Cross-promotion is a great way to broaden your reach and to allow for different types of interaction. Eventually you might even find that you do significantly better on one platform over another. Cross-promotion also bolsters your SEO game, because it means that you own more online real estate.

Cross-Posting Is Not Cross-Promoting

Instagram has an option for people to share points directly to Facebook or Twitter from Instagram. But when you do this, hashtags carry over, which you definitely don't want on Facebook. Tags don't carry over. When the post goes over to Twitter, you'll lose the imagery and lose the engagement to go with it.

When you cross-post, you're sharing the same exact post on every social media platform without changing the captain length, the image formatting, vocabulary, tags, or anything else. It means you're automatically sharing a post that's meant for Twitter and will not resonate with Facebook followers (or be formatted for the platform). Cross-posting runs the risk of losing the audience's attention, and it might make you look a little lazy.

Each social media site has different best practices, different formats, and even different times of day that's best to post. You want to change it up for each platform.

If this sounds like a lot of work, it's not. All you have to do is slightly change the delivery of the same message. Most of the time, all it takes are tiny tweaks here and there that make a post more appropriate for the specific social media site it's destined for. A post on Instagram will look pretty different than the same content on LinkedIn.

Useful Tools

Having the right tools makes content creation so much easier. Design beautiful graphics in a flash, check your grammar, grain valuable insight from your audience, and create your very own GIFs. Here are just a few of the best creative tools that the best content creators swear by.

Hashtagify.me

On Twitter and Instagram, hashtags can represent the difference between hundreds of people seeing your post, and, well, nobody seeing your post. Hashtagify helps you drive up engagement by ensuring that you're using the most used, popular hashtags. It helps you check what hashtags the top influencers are using in your field, helps you choose the hashtags that work best for you, and gives you insights to boost your performance and drive engagement.

SlideShare and SlideSnack

SlideShare, powered by LinkedIn, is a great way for professionals to share their presentations, infographics, documents, or videos from which other professionals can view and learn. It's a great way to share your research and knowledge with other professionals in your field and also allows you to easily view presentations from other experts. For many, it's easier to absorb the information from a visual SlideShare deck than from a dense study.

SlideSnack is another presentation-sharing tool that enables you to easily upload and share presentations online. On SlideSnack, you can record presentations and export video, making it easy to share presentations on your website, blog, YouTube, or social media channels.

Grammarly

If you're writing anything online, you might benefit from an editor. Grammarly edits your copy for you to ensure that you don't publish anything with embarrassing typos or mistakes. Grammarly doesn't just check grammar and spelling mistakes, though. They take it a step further by suggesting words, pointing out passive voice, and ensuring that your content has good readability and flow.

Giphy

We all love GIFs – those short, moving images that are so effective in cracking a joke or making your content stand out with color and movement. It's a short video that repeats over and over again, and Giphy is your go-to for the most popular and newest GIFs, and you can also make your own.

Vidyard

Vidyard kicks the power of video up a notch by providing users with the insights they need to improve their video strategy. They help video producers and marketers capture a viewer's attention within the first few seconds, close a video effectively, and include calls-to-action in their videos.

SurveyMonkey

For those with an already-established audience, sometimes it's good to know how you're doing, what your audience thinks, and what they want to see more of (and less of!) in the future. With SurveyMonkey, you can easily develop your own online surveys that you can share across your platforms, so you can connect with your audience and hear what they think in their own words.

Anchor

Anchor is a podcasting tool for beginners. Their tagline is "the easiest way to start a podcast." On this easy and free platform, you can record high-quality audio or upload audio of your own, host an unlimited amount of episodes, and distribute your episodes across your social media platforms.

Typeform

Typeform is a data collection tool that helps you gather data from your audience that can inform your content creation decisions moving forward. Like SurveyMonkey, you can easily create surveys, polls, and quizzes. But it doesn't stop there. Make contact forms, online shop pages, landing pages, and customer feedback forms that look great and are easy to use.

Typorama

Typorama is a free graphics tool that helps you easily design beautiful social media graphics, choose typography for your images, crop images, and share to your social media sites with ease.

Animoto

Animoto provides a way to easily make video out of photos, video clips, and music so you can stand out on social media. Video creation and editing can be highly time-consuming, and Animoto seeks to cut out some of that time and effort.

Placeit

Placeit is perfect if you need a logo but don't want to pay the hundreds of dollars you'll pay to hire a designer for a custom one. With Placeit, you can create logos, videos, designs, and mockups cheaply and simply. You can even make tee shirts and desktop backgrounds.

Canva

Canva is a popular go-to for easily creating social media graphics. It makes graphic design approachable and easy. Create stunning Instagram posts, postcards, business cards, flyers, invitations, Facebook covers, Facebook posts, Twitter posts, Twitter covers, photo collages, blog banners, and much more.

Hootsuite

If you need a center-of-the-wheel for your multiple social media sites, then consider looking into Hootsuite. Hootsuite helps you manage multiple social media networks, measure your impact on each, schedule posts on each platform, and track return of investment.

Role Models of Content Creation

Sometimes the most powerful inspiration comes from admiring other people's work. Through the example of others, we can get a sense for what works, how physicians maintain a thread of consistency throughout their content, and what creative liberties reward them with engagement.

Dr. Howard Luks

An orthopedic surgeon who specializes in shoulder, knee, and other sports injuries, Dr. Howard Luks is a content creator extraordinaire. He focuses his energy on blogging and YouTube videos, where he educates athletes about everything related to sports injuries – from how to tell if you have a serious injury, to exercise best practices, to essentials for speedy recovery. On YouTube, his videos skew on the short side, ranging anywhere from 1 to 10 minutes. Mostly, his videos are of him sharing his professional opinion in front of the camera – nothing too intricate – but one of his videos about meniscal tears has been viewed almost 200,000 times.

Dr. Sandra Lee (aka Dr. Pimple Popper)

Dr. Lee's most successful platform is no doubt her YouTube page, which boasts no less than four million subscribers. The dermatologist, skin cancer surgeon, and cosmetic surgeon shares videos about common skin issues and cutting-edge cosmetic surgery techniques and practices. Her content is incredibly consistent – her videos are always procedure-focused and show viewers the "how" behind dermatology.

New York Dynamic Neuromuscular Rehabilitation

A physical therapy clinic that specializes in neuromuscular rehabilitation, New York Dynamic Neuromuscular Rehab, generates much of their own content to show off their state-of-the-art facilities, common physical therapy procedures, and inspirational quotes. Their content is so original, in fact, that they don't share anything that *isn't* original. They share upcoming events and workshops, self-published blog posts, and visual information regarding physical therapy.

Dr. Wendy Sue Swanson (Seattle Mama Doc)

I previously mentioned Dr. Wendy Sue Swanson in Chap. 7 because of the thoughtful way she shares external, non-original articles from trustworthy news outlets. But when she does create her own content, she allows followers to see a glimpse of her own life "behind the scenes," which makes her appear warm, genuine, and an ally to the parents who turn to her for relevant information about child health.

Seattle Mama Doc writes her own blog posts and records her own podcasts and videos. She stays timely, both with relevant health news and seasonal disease information to keep her patients informed. She often dispels common health myths: such as fruit juice being a "go-to" for toddlers (she says the sugar content is too high), educates about drowning prevention, and much more.

Dr. Swanson is a perfect example of how using multiple platforms can strengthen your message and help you reach broader audiences. She's on Twitter, Facebook, and runs a blog and podcast. She's in a lot of places at once. And she keeps things interesting by differentiating her content across platforms.

Be Careful! A Word of Caution

As physicians, we have a higher responsibility than most people when it comes to our social media use. On a weekly basis, we're privy to the private information of hundreds of patients. Maintaining a public image of utmost professionalism is essential. A single slipup could result in a loss of trust among your patients and damage your professional reputation. Here are some important rules to keep in mind before you hit the "publish" button.

You might be surprised at how easy it can be to violate patient privacy. Some physicians violate privacy online without even realizing they caused a problem. Know the sneaky signs. According to a review conducted by the Veterans Affairs Medical Center in Washington, DC, violating patient privacy is easier than one might think [10].

Rule of thumb: never post any information, comments, photos, or videos concerning a patient to a social networking site. If you must share patient stories, make sure that nobody could identify the patient, and when in doubt, always get permission. While writing about patients, privacy can become a difficult issue to navigate. According to a study that reviewed 271 medical blogs written by healthcare professionals and physicians, individual patients were described in 42% of the samples. Seventeen percent included enough information for patients to identify themselves or their providers, and three included recognizable photographs of their patients [11].

Your social media presence should illuminate your skills, knowledge, and professionalism, not make you liable under HIPAA and state privacy laws!

Sometimes, patient privacy is violated in more blatant ways. In 2013, a doctor posted pictures of a young female patient hooked up to an IV after an episode of binge drinking. He posted these pictures, with a comment about her condition, without consent from the patient. That patient sued Northwestern University Hospital $1.5 million in damages [12].

In Georgia, a dermatologist who practiced as a cosmetic surgeon uploaded multiple videos of herself dancing around her clinic while performing surgery. She claimed that these videos were consensual from the patients, but that didn't help her in court when multiple patients came forward to raise major malpractice concerns. The videos – and the disfigurement of her patients – resulted in a 2.5 year suspension of her medical license [13].

So, be smart. When you create your own content on social media, make sure it's in good taste and reflects how you want to be seen as a professional. Here are some good ways to scan whether a post is appropriate before you post it:

- Perform an emotional appeal check
Read your post with fresh eyes. Will it have the intended emotional reaction you're going for? If you're not sure, then step back and wait a day before posting it. If you're still not sure, don't post it at all.

- Edit your work
Always look over your work to ensure that you're not about to make a slipup that could make you look unprofessional. This goes for grammar, too!

The Difference Between Good and Great Content

Great content gets more shares and engagement and can have a major impact on how patients and other healthcare professionals perceive you. Here are some tips to make your page stand out, to gain followers, and to keep the ones you already have engaged.

- *Don't forget to tag the people you mentioned or quoted in your blog posts*
And that doesn't just go for blog posts. If you're posting a colleague's study, sharing a podcast from a doctor you admire in Baltimore, or mention someone in a video, be sure to tag that person. With every person tagged, more people see the post, which leads to a spike in engagement.

- *Use hashtags so people can find you*
We don't use hashtags on every social networking platform; they're unnecessary on Facebook and LinkedIn, for example. But on Twitter and Instagram, you're going to want to use hashtags. For example, if your post is about the most recent findings concerning pregnancy nutrition, some ideal hashtags might be: #pregnancynutrition, #OBGYN, #pregnancy, #newmoms, and the like. (Be sure to use Hashtagify.me to find the strongest hashtags for any given post!)

- *Listen to feedback*
There are several ways to get feedback from readers. You can ask questions in your posts or create polls or surveys. Listening to feedback can inform how you

create content moving forward – what resonates with your followers, what doesn't, what they care about, what they're anxious about, what questions they have, and what they want to see more of from you.

- *Don't be afraid to get funny or personal*
Dr. Dave Stukus (@AllergyKidsDoc) is a perfect example of how a little bit of humor can help you connect with audiences. By sharing funny GIFs along with valuable medical information, he's catching and keeping the interest of his followers and adding a human touch to a topic that could be sterile and impersonal.

And speaking of personal, it's absolutely okay to share what you believe, pictures from your vacation in France, the bittersweet sadness you might feel on your kids' first day of school, or to snap a selfie of yourself on the plane as you're headed to a conference. These glimpses of everyday life allow patients to get to know you and to potentially feel more at home with you when they meet you in the exam room.

- *Thank your followers*
A little bit of gratitude goes a long way. When you hit 500, 1000, and other major follower milestones, send out a good, hearty thanks to the people who follow you.

- *Stay consistent and post regularly*
You'll find that it's harder to post on some weeks than others. You might run out of content sometimes. You might just be too darn busy. But a good rule of thumb is to ensure that you post at least three times a week. Many social media experts say that you should post every single day – sometimes twice a day – but just do what you can.

In order to stay consistent, refer back to your content strategy, and consider how each blog article, podcast, or social post you send out into the world is strongly related to your specialty or niche.

- *Keep your content brief and to the point*
When followers see a wall of text, they're likely to keep scrolling. People typically don't have time to sit and read a novel on Facebook. Make sure that you're communicating the most important points up front and combing through your content to ensure that you don't ramble on.

- *Aesthetics matter, so take your time and make everything look professional*
A professional-looking website will support people's perception of you as a professional. Just as a beautiful, state-of-the-art hospital makes patients feel like they'll get the best care, a professional website, beautiful posts, and a high-quality standard for content will add to your perceived expertise.

- *Use statistics: Know when to post, who you're posting to, what performs well, and what doesn't*

On Facebook, the "Insights" tab in your page is a goldmine of valuable information. For everything else, there's Typeform so you can dive into the statistics that will drive your messaging. With the use of statistics, you can get valuable insight on who your audience is (the real people might be different than who you expected to attract!), when they're online, and which posts perform the best overall.

See How You're Doing: Analyzing Social Media Statistics

When you have your social media insights at your fingertips, there's no reason to not use them. Social media insights can improve your messaging, help you create content that resonates with your followers, and increase your engagement. It can help you know when your followers are online so you can get more eyes on your posts. It can help you see the long term of which types of posts performed poorly and which types of posts skyrocketed in engagement. The results might surprise you!

Here are some essential statistics that can help you improve your content creation strategy:

Page Views

Page views are useful when you want to see how many unique visitors click over to your page. This can let in you in on a powerful secret: which content is so compelling that it's making people stop in their tracks and click over to your page?

Organic Likes and Traffic

If you don't want to pay Facebook to launch an ad campaign, then you're going to have to rely on organic likes. Organic traffic refers to the amount of people who have engaged with your posts and liked your page – without being pulled in from paid advertisements. This is an important distinction, because when people begin following your page naturally, it means that they deem your content compelling enough to want to see more.

Conversion Rates

If you're trying to get people on Facebook to go check out your podcast or if you're trying to get Instagram followers to read your blog, analytics can show you who clicked your call to action. It can show you how many people, from which platforms, took the action you wanted them to. For this, Google Analytics is best.

Engagement Rates

Engagement rates refer to the number of people that interact with your content through likes, comments, or shares. This is especially useful when looking at your posts over time. You might realize that your audience doesn't really care about podcasts but absolutely loves it when you post inspirational quotes. Or, you might find that your audience doesn't engage as much when you share research, but they really engage when you share behind-the-scenes pictures of life at the hospital.

Audience Growth

Audience growth refers to the new subscribers or leads that are generated from a piece of content. This helps you recognize whether your content has been attracting new people or turning people away. Over the long term, you'll be able to tell what kind of content loses people and what content brings more to your page. You can see audience growth by day and, perhaps more tellingly, when you lost followers.

Demographic Metrics

How old are your followers? Are they mostly male or female? Do they live in the American south, or all they mostly concentrated on the west coast? On LinkedIn, you can even see what positions people hold. Are your followers managers, directors, or mainly entry-level workers? This helps you understand how your content resonates with different audiences and ensures that you're attracting the right people.

There are some great analytics tools out there to help make this process quicker and easier.

Google Analytics

Google Analytics is so robust that there's not much it can't tell you. This powerful analytics tool can even tell you which social media sites are the most effective for you. It can tell you which social media sites attract people to your website, get people to sign up for your newsletter, and how long those people stay on your website, blog, or podcast landing page.

Sprout Social

Sprout is another great tool. It not only helps you manage your multiple social media accounts, but it can show you which hashtags perform the best, how you're doing compared to others in your field, and even gain insight on how people are talking about you on Twitter.

Using the statistics at your fingertips is a surefire way to ensure that you're spending your energy where you're going to get the biggest return on investment. It ensures that you're posting in the right place, at the right time, and attracting the right audience. It can help you see which social media behaviors positively impact your bottom line – whether that bottom line is to attract new patients, get people listening to your podcast, or get more reads on your healthcare blog.

Conclusion

Creating your own content can be incredibly rewarding. It can give you a yearbook-style history on how far you've come in your personal career or practice. It can give you the clarity to better know who you are as a healthcare provider and give you valuable insight on the patients that step into your office every day. As more and more people – and medical professionals – are logging onto social media platforms to learn, engage, and gather together with their online communities, professionals can carve a place for themselves where they can educate, dispel myths, and arm their patients with the knowledge they need to improve the health outcomes in their lives.

References

1. Hamilton, K. 30 amazing mobile health technology statistics for today's physician. ReferralMD, 18 Nov 2017, getreferralmd.com/2015/08/mobile-healthcare-technology-statistics/.
2. Weaver J. More people search for health online. NBCNews.com, NBCUniversal News Group, 16 July 2003, www.nbcnews.com/id/3077086/t/more-people-search-health-online/#. W7K8yVPwZYc.
3. Patel N. 38 content marketing stats that every marketer needs to know. Neil Patel, 3 July 2018, neilpatel.com/blog/38-content-marketing-stats-that-every-marketer-needs-to-know/.
4. The nine ingredients that make great content. Neil Patel, 12 July 2018, neilpatel.com/blog/ingredients-of-great-content/.
5. Strong E. Strong medicine. YouTube, www.youtube.com/channel/UCFq5vPnNRNNN ysLrktz4aSw.
6. 27 video stats for 2017 | 2017 media statistics – Insivia. Insivia Marketing Web Design, 26 Sept 2018, www.insivia.com/27-video-stats-2017/.
7. Maria J. 45 video marketing statistics. Virtuets, www.virtuets.com/45-video-marketing-statistics/.
8. Knott J. 20 incredible medical marketing statistics. Intrepy Healthcare Marketing, 21 July 2018, intrepy.com/20-incredible-medical-marketing-statistics/.
9. Patrick M. A pediatric podcast for parents. PediaCast, Nationwide Children's Hospital, 2018., www.pediacast.org/.
10. Chretien KC, Kind T. Social media and clinical care: ethical, professional, and social implications. Curr Neurol Neurosci Rep, US National Library of Medicine, 2 Apr 2013., www.ncbi.nlm.nih.gov/pubmed/23547180/.

11. Ventola CL. Social media and health care professionals: benefits, risks, and best practices. Curr Neurol Neurosci Rep, U.S. National Library of Medicine, July 2014., www.ncbi.nlm.nih.gov/pmc/articles/PMC4103576/.
12. Woman sues Northwestern after doctor posted drunk photos. CBS Chicago, CBS Chicago, 21 Aug 2013., chicago.cbslocal.com/2013/08/21/woman-sues-northwestern-after-doctor-posted-drunk-photos/.
13. Ellis R, Lynch J. 'Dancing Doctor' agrees to two-and-a-half-year suspension of medical license, records show. CNN, Cable News Network, 1 July 2018, www.cnn.com/2018/06/29/us/dancing-doctor-medical-license/index.html.

Dos and Don'ts: Social Media Tips for the Medical Professional

9

Diane Davis Lang

When angry, count to four. When very angry, swear.

—Mark Twain

Social Media Policy

Social media platforms are spaces where individuals can connect with friends and peers and where medical professionals can speak to their knowledge, passion, and service. Much as previous generations talked over fences or on front porches, social media allows users to connect about the latest news in their neighborhoods and all around the world. A well-run social media account injects personality in a conversational tone to engage with community in an authentic way. This authenticity means users sometimes let their guards down and open up their innermost thoughts to friends, fans, and followers. This is definitely okay to do; the best social media users are individuals and entities who make a personal connection with their audience, but this freedom of sharing can cause users to post content that could be detrimental to themselves or their organization.

A social media policy serves many purposes, but its most important role is to ensure that the use of social media does not jeopardize compliance with laws and regulations or compromise confidential and proprietary information. Healthcare companies should adhere to this policy for official organizational use of social media. Organizational use is defined as any use of social media for the purpose of (1) representing or appearing to represent the views, positions, or statements of an organization; (2) creating or posting to online forums, social media accounts, blogs, or other applications which provide access to information about the organization; and (3) performing job responsibilities through social media. To put it simply, this policy serves as a reminder to act in a professional and compliant manner when posting to social media platforms on an organization's behalf.

© Springer Nature Switzerland AG 2019
D. R. Stukus et al., *Social Media for Medical Professionals*,
https://doi.org/10.1007/978-3-030-14439-5_9

However, a social media policy should not just be limited to organizational use. These guidelines should be practiced by anyone who has affiliated themselves with the organization, both online and offline, including all employees, trainees, and volunteers. This includes the use of social media for nonprofessional purposes or for purposes that are unrelated to an employee's association with their organization. Just as someone would not stand on a public street doing something that could jeopardize their career, they should not post content online that could do the same. A good rule of thumb is to pretend the CEO is always watching! If a business has a social media policy, it is best practice for the employees of that business to follow the policy guidelines whether they are sharing the latest research or a picture of their pet. A social media policy assures that content is not offensive and serves as a reminder that a user's actions can reflect upon their organization's reputation. Not to mention, poor use could hinder career growth and momentum.

Confidentiality

Patients and their families trust medical professionals with private information ranging from lab results to financial information. Maintaining that confidentiality is not only good business practice; it is the law. By ensuring that an individual's identifiable health information is protected, the HIPAA Privacy Rule gives clear guidelines on organizational compliance and the use of patient data. The Privacy Rule protects healthcare systems from fraud and gives patients the right to privacy. The use of patient information on social media, including images, names, diagnosis, or treatment, is only allowed if there is signed HIPAA consent or de-identified information. De-identification is the process of removing details that could identify a patient.

This confidentiality should be the cornerstone of any healthcare social media policy. For the sake of sharing on social media, we will consider the "Safe Harbor" method of de-identification from the US Department of Health and Human Services. This means making patients anonymous by removing Private Health Information (PHI), which is a set of 18 criteria including [1]:

- Names
- All geographic subdivisions smaller than a state, including street address, city, county, precinct, zip code, and their equivalent geocodes, except for the initial three digits of the zip code if, according to the current publicly available data from the Bureau of the Census:
  1. The geographic unit formed by combining all zip codes with the same three initial digits contains more than 20,000 people.
  2. The initial three digits of a zip code for all such geographic units containing 20,000 or fewer people are changed to 000.
- All elements of dates (except year) for dates that are directly related to an individual, including birth date, admission date, discharge date, death date, and all ages over 89 and all elements of dates (including year) indicative of such age,

except that such ages and elements may be aggregated into a single category of age 90 or older
- Telephone numbers
- Vehicle identifiers and serial numbers, including license plate numbers
- Fax numbers
- Device identifiers and serial numbers
- Email addresses
- Web Universal Resource Locators (URLs)
- Social security numbers
- Internet Protocol (IP) addresses
- Medical record numbers
- Biometric identifiers, including finger and voice prints
- Health plan beneficiary numbers
- Full-face photographs and any comparable images
- Account numbers
- Any other unique identifying number, characteristic, or code
- Certificate/license numbers

How can a user decide if the patient information is identifiable? Principles used by experts in the determination of the identifiability of health information from the US Department of Health and Human Services include replicability, data source availability, distinguishability, and risk assessment [2] (Table 9.1).

Twitter chats, Instagram, Facebook Live, or Facebook Groups can be great ways to engage with other clinicians to discuss cases or research, but when posting photographs or discussing diagnoses on social media, users must take care not to include PHI in their posts. This is accomplished by de-identifying content to assure that all PHI has been removed. The public nature of social media and its high data source availability makes identification a higher concern. Physicians who work within a small geographic area, with a small demographic (i.e., pediatricians in a rural area), have a greater chance that cases can be identified. Those chances greatly increase when shared on an international social media platform. The US Department of Health and Human Services estimates that the combination of a patient's date of birth, gender, and 5-digit zip code is unique for over 50% of residents in the United States. Those three criteria in combination have the potential to identify half of the country's population. When sharing case studies, it is best to stick to broad, general terms, conditions, and age ranges (Fig. 9.1).

Social media usage also has unique risks outside of medical case studies. As the age demographic of medical professionals gets younger, social media usage by employees is getting more active and broad. With 78% of 18- to 24-year-olds using Snapchat and 71% using Instagram [3], hospitals and healthcare organizations are at risk simply by the nature of a younger workforce and their affinity for social media tools and engagement. Social media users may share photos of themselves in public spaces and may not realize there are identifying factors all around, including patients, families, or other PHI in the background. While many organizations encourage staff social media engagement for brand elevation, users should be

Table 9.1 Factors that determine whether something contains any identifiable information

Principle	Description	Examples
Replicability	Prioritize health information features into levels of risk according to the chance it will consistently occur in relation to the individual	*Low replicability*: Results of a patient's blood glucose level test will vary *High replicability*: Demographics of a patient (e.g., birth date) are relatively stable
Data source availability	Determine which external data sources contain the patients' identifiers and the replicable features in the health information, as well as who is permitted access to the data source	*Low data source availability*: The results of laboratory reports are not often disclosed with identity beyond healthcare environments *High data source availability*: Patient name and demographics are often in public data sources, such as vital records – Birth, death, and marriage registries
Distinguishability	Determine the extent to which the subject's data can be distinguished in the health information	*Low distinguishability*: It has been estimated that the combination of *year of birth*, *gender*, and *3-digit zip code* is unique for approximately 0.04% of residents in the United States. This means that very few residents could be identified through this combination of data alone *High distinguishability*: It has been estimated that the combination of a patient's *date of birth*, *gender*, and *5-digit zip code* is unique for over 50% of residents in the United States. This means that over half of US residents could be uniquely described just with these three data elements
Assess risk	The greater the replicability, availability, and distinguishability of the health information, the greater the risk for identification	*Low risk assessment*: Laboratory values may be very distinguishing, but they are rarely independently replicable and are rarely disclosed in multiple data sources to which many people have access *High risk assessment*: Demographics are highly distinguishing, highly replicable, and available in public data sources

instructed to be diligent about what is included in photos. This could include a license plate of a car outside of a hospital or a whiteboard in the background of staff photo. Staff should be trained and frequently reminded to be mindful of the types of content they are sharing and told that PHI must always be protected.

Disclosing Intellectual Property, Fair Use, and Creative Commons

One of the first lessons we are taught as students is to keep our eyes on our own paper. Copying may be considered a form of flattery, but it can also be considered a violation of copyright law. When sharing online content, it is always in a

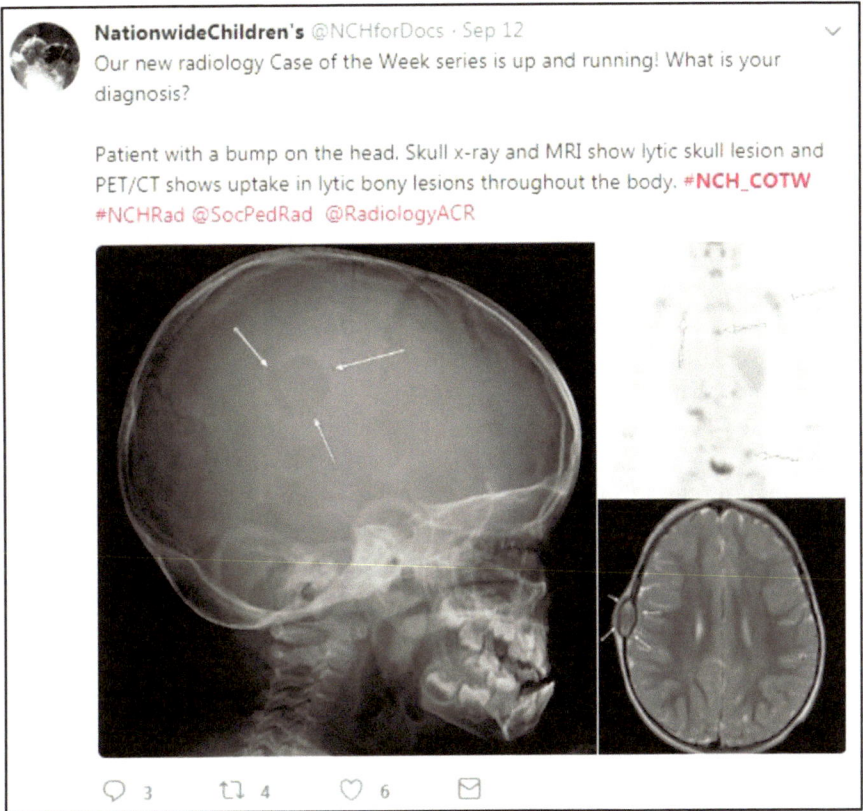

NationwideChildren's @NCHforDocs · Sep 12
Our new radiology Case of the Week series is up and running! What is your diagnosis?

Patient with a bump on the head. Skull x-ray and MRI show lytic skull lesion and PET/CT shows uptake in lytic bony lesions throughout the body. **#NCH_COTW** #NCHRad @SocPedRad @RadiologyACR

3   4   6

Fig. 9.1 Example of a Twitter post with de-identified information. (Adapted from https://twitter.com/NCHforDocs)

user's best interest to seek permission from the original creator, and this process should be reflected in an organization's social media policy. However, as social media continues to evolve, so do the rules of copyright surrounding its use. "Fair use" states that the use of work for purposes that include criticism, comment, teaching, or research is not a form of copyright infringement – all of which can be considered forms of social media expression. When reproducing work under fair use, the following, outlined in the Copyright Act of 1976, should be considered [4]:

- The purpose and character of the use, including whether such use is of a commercial nature or is for nonprofit educational purposes
- The nature of the copyrighted work
- The amount of the portion used in relation to the copyrighted work as a whole
- The effect of the use upon the potential market for or value of the copyrighted work

Somewhat outside the realm of federal copyright law sits the international non-profit organization, Creative Commons, which allows Internet users to share and repurpose online material. With more than 1.4 billion pieces of content [5], Creative Commons allows social media users to publish and share content with some limitations. Among other things, Creative Commons licenses allow licensees to:

- Copy the work
- Distribute the work
- Edit the work
- Display the work publicly
- Use the work digitally

As a Creative Commons content creator, users can restrict how content is republished and how those pieces of content are attributed. This could mean requiring someone to link to an original piece of work, keep it marked with a copyright, or ensure full restrictions by not allowing changes to the content or licensing. This open concept allows social media users a great deal of freedom when searching for, or sharing, content. The licenses fall under the categories outlined in Table 9.2 [6].

Table 9.2 Creative Commons licenses

License	Cite origin	Noncommercial	Commercial	Derivative licensure
Attribution	X	X	X	
Attribution-ShareAlike	X	X	X	X
Attribution-NoDerivs	X	X	X	
Attribution-NonCommercial	X	X		
Attribution-NonCommercial-ShareAlike	X	X	X	X
Attribution-NonCommercial-NoDerivs	X	X		

Attribution – This allows users to share and alter content as long as the original creator is cited. This license applies to commercial use as well as noncommercial.

Attribution-ShareAlike – This license allows users to share and alter content as long as the original creator is cited and the original Creative Commons license follows any derivative works.

Attribution-NoDerivs – This license allows users to share unaltered content as long as the original creator is cited.

Attribution-NonCommercial – This license allows users to share and alter content as long as the original creator is cited. It is not for commercial use, and the original Creative Commons license does not follow derivative works.

Attribution-NonCommercial-ShareAlike – This license allows users to share and alter content as long as the original creator is cited. It is not for commercial use, and the original Creative Commons license follows all derivative works.

Attribution-NonCommercial-NoDerivs – This license allows users to share work as long as the original creator is cited. The content cannot be used commercially nor can it be altered in any way.

Photos and Videos

Creative Commons provides social media users with numerous options for curating and repurposing images and infographics – which is a best practice in the realm of social media. Photos and videos increase engagement by up to 85% on Facebook, alone [7], and users are encouraged to include a visual asset in every shared post, no matter the social media platform. This can include images of patients, their families, their pathologies, and radiologic images. If these images include patient information or their likeness, a signed HIPAA consent form should be obtained, and the patient, or their parent or guardian, must agree to each piece of private information that may be disclosed, including but not limited to name, age, diagnosis, and treatment. The authorization should also include information about where the photo or video will be shared, acknowledgment that the image is public and must disclose the purpose of sharing. It should also note whether the consent pertains to news media and how long the permission will be in effect. Without signed HIPAA consent, the image must be de-identified. Obtaining signed HIPAA consent may seem like a barrier to sharing, but it is a necessary one. Moreover, by putting in the extra effort on the front end, engagement will likely increase on the back end.

Threats and False Statements

It is easy to be pulled into conversations with users on social media who may have differing views – some of whom have extremely vocal opinions. You will learn more about these users or trolls in Chap. 10. Trolls, for the most part, do not care about facts or evidence-based information or practices, and medical professionals should take care in addressing them. Engaging with trolls can lead even the most seasoned and professional social media user to make mistakes and get involved in conversations that could easily end up damaging a reputation. Healthcare professionals on social media should keep content factual and should not use inflammatory language in addressing users. Better yet, it is best to ignore them entirely. Many of these situations can be quelled by avoiding engagement with those who fall to one extreme or another in their opinion. Certain topics are known to increase radical reactions in healthcare social media. Vaccinations and animal testing may be imperative to public health and research, but do not tend to bring out moderate users on social media.

If a user feels threatened by a social media post, the first thing they should do is take a screenshot of the content. Threats should then be reported to the social media platform, the user's legal department – if posting on behalf of an organization – and, based on the level of the threat, possibly the authorities. The social media platform, like Facebook or Twitter, may also alert authorities, but the rules enforced through their community guidelines can be fluid and ever changing. It is in the user's best interest to be proactive and vigilant in ignoring and blocking any threatening behavior of which they are aware.

Fig. 9.2 Example of potential defamation on Twitter. (Adapted from https://twitter.com/realDonaldTrump)

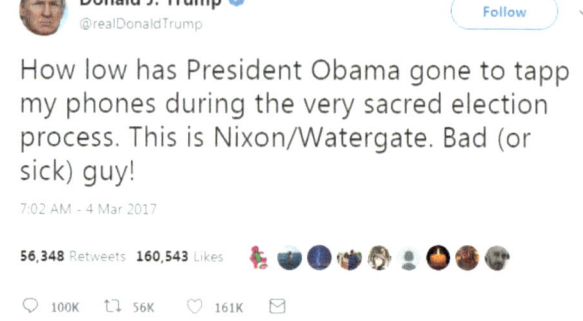

Harassment or Defamation

Merriam-Webster defines defamation as the act of communicating false statements about a person that injures the reputation of that person. Look closely at a politician's or religious leader's Twitter feed and the users with whom they engage, and you will probably find examples of borderline, or blatant, harassment and defamation. The examples are everywhere, including the highest political office in the world. In March 2017, US President Donald Trump came under fire for tweets which were potentially libelous against former US President Barack Obama [8] (Fig. 9.2).

If Obama had chosen to proceed with a lawsuit claiming this wiretapping statement was false, could it be ascertained that the statement was communicated? Probably so. Not only was it published on a public platform from a public account, but it was shared over 56,000 times by other Twitter users. Though state laws vary, if it were determined that Obama's reputation had been harmed because of this statement, and if Trump had not been a sitting president at the time, he could have been open to litigation. The office of the president protects the sitting President from civil lawsuits, but the average citizen docs not wield that power [6, 9]. In order to protect reputations, users should not make accusations, nor should they allow them to be made about them.

Explicit Content

Though it seems like common sense, people have certainly been terminated for their social media use. In order to uphold professionalism and refrain from damaging their own reputation or that of their institution, social media users should never post obscene or profane content. Posts that contain sexual references or references to illegal drug use are examples of the kind of thing that is best kept off social media. Users should never use language that would be unacceptable in the workplace, paying special attention not to disparage any race, religion, gender, sexual orientation, disability, or national origin. This includes linking to, or referring to, sites that contain maliciously false, harassing, pornographic, or indecent content. Remember, what one person thinks is funny or ironic may not be to someone else.

These rules do not only apply when an employee is on the clock. It is not uncommon for concerned social media users or patients to make organizations aware of their staff's social media use via screenshots or links sent by private message, email, or a compliance hotline. This includes their activities outside of working hours. Even if the content does not violate an organization's social media policy, co-workers, managers, friends, and even family members can use social media posts in vengeful ways or as retaliation. At times, users are lulled into a false sense of security by posting in private groups or on platforms like Snapchat, a mobile application that allows users to send photos that "disappear" after being viewed. However, it is entirely a possibility that someone can take a screenshot of any online image – even from another device – and reshare it. Private or closed social media groups and accounts do not afford a user any more privacy than a public space when a screenshot is simply a click away.

Endorsements

A diverse and inclusive workforce is comprised of many different views and opinions, and healthcare workers are, by nature, advocates for physical and mental health. While these advocates should be encouraged to affiliate themselves with their organization and share vibrant and unique perspectives, endorsements in conjunction with their job title can be considered promotional and cause tax implications. Healthcare facilities operating as nonprofits, and their faculty and staff acting on the organization's behalf, should follow 501(c)(3) regulations and should not endorse any product, candidate, or cause in affiliation with their job title. Although it would have to be proven that the reference was an inducement to make a purchase and the post would need to be a substantial benefit to the corporation whose product was endorsed, it is best practice to refrain from mentioning brands. Thanking corporate sponsors for support of a nonprofit should not result in tax implications, but delving into product endorsements may be considered advertising. This risk increases with the mention of cost, checkout, or purchasing products. Maintaining appropriate advertising boundaries means giving no inducement to purchase or use products or services, Fig. 9.3. These guidelines also extend to the endorsement of political issues, candidates, or causes.

Fig. 9.3 A physician can recommend the use of ibuprofen but would want to avoid brand names when making the recommendation on social media

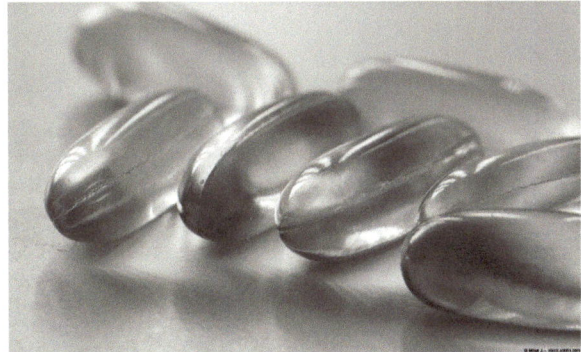

Conducting Business on Social Media

As social media use becomes more prolific, many consumers have an expectation that they will get questions answered, or their concerns addressed, immediately. While it is certainly acceptable for many companies to conduct business via social media, a designated entity or department who has permission to do so should publish and monitor the content. Healthcare professionals who may be perceived as speaking on behalf of their organization should be aware of community guidelines and organizational protocols. Medical advice provided should be general and linked to evidence-based resources or guidelines. When a social media user asks questions that a healthcare worker cannot answer by linking to resources, the reply should include the recommendation that the patient be seen by their primary care physician. To maintain professionalism, healthcare providers should never conduct official business or perform job responsibilities through social media. This pleads the case for organizations to have robust online content with thorough resources for patients. With 80% of Internet users looking online for healthcare information [10], a well-designed website with accurate and evidence-based information can provide answers to questions while keeping users in a funnel to drive revenue and referrals [11]. Whether the patient is in need of an answer to how to ease cold symptoms, looking for a specialist or wanting to know directions to a location, a well-designed website or digital application can help them find the answers and keep them engaged in the organization's content.

Media Relations

One of the most satisfying aspects of healthcare social media is making a difference to public health by disseminating evidence-based information to those who need it. Think of parents who are comforting a crying baby in the middle of the night, a patient who feels scary physical symptoms when they are away from home or the people who simply do not have access to health care services. All of them are examples of people who might be looking online for healthcare information, and sometimes a post will resonate with large groups of people. Stories and posts that reach mass interest can draw attention from reporters, podcasters, and bloggers. Without a public relations team at the ready, this can be intimidating. However, with the right knowledge and preparation, media relations can be an extension of the advocacy done by healthcare professionals on social media. News media earned by socially savvy healthcare professionals may come as a result of speaking out or sharing content about unique services, treatments, research, or trending news stories. Unlike what we would have seen a generation ago, reporters now scroll through Twitter feeds looking for expert opinions on the latest news. This is another reason to always share fact-based content on social media. Doing so assures that a reporter has the correct information before reaching out and the healthcare professional is represented fairly as a trusted resource. Recognize that any engagement done on social media is considered "on the record" by reporters. Users should always err on the side of caution and non-disclosure of PHI, and HIPAA consent should still be top of mind.

Speaking on Behalf of the Organization

Media reach out is not the only way in which medical professionals represent their organization. Medical professionals may choose to share content as a business entity instead of using a personal account. Social media accounts affiliated with an organization should have a clear disclaimer and community guidelines which address account moderation frequency and what constitutes the need for guideline enforcement. What type of content would your organization deem inappropriate enough to hide, delete, or block? These community guidelines should address:

- Comment deletion policy (i.e., hate speech, profanity, vulgarity, obscenity)
- Deletion or blocking of community members
- Nudity
- Defamation, name calling, or personal attacks
- Comments that violate privacy of patients or their families
- Promotional comments, including promotion of events, products, groups, pages, websites, or programs not affiliated with the organization
- The right to repost or reproduce content
- Statement that nothing posted should be considered medical advice
- Age guidelines
- Anything else the page, group, or account moderator deems inappropriate

Employees posting from a personal account, or to an organization's affiliated account, should follow the guidelines of the organization's social media policy. An affiliated business account has the additional duty of following and enforcing the community guidelines.

Complaint Protocol

Having a professional persona on social media, either as a business or as an individual, means there will come a time to face detractors. Detractors in healthcare mostly consist of people who have had bad experiences or who disagree with business practices. This can mean everything from office hours and wait times to diagnosis and follow-up. Having a complaint protocol in place makes it easy to maintain composure when reacting. This protocol does not have to be lengthy and complex but rather quick, short, and non-incendiary with matter of fact language that helps the user see that action is being taken to address their complaint. The protocol should have the following components:

- Acknowledge the complaint.
- Ask to have them send additional feedback, comments, or information to an email account or via phone call.
- Escalate, if necessary, to patient relations team, manager, public relations, or legal teams
- Do not respond to trolls.

The best option for responding to a complaint is to take the conversation offline. It is quite easy for users in a social media thread to take on a hive mind and make a conversation escalate into an angry venue where all detractors dump their thoughts. Acknowledging the comment and letting detractors know they are heard are often all they want. By requesting follow-up, either by email or a phone call, also reinforces marketing engagement strategy and lets the community at large know there is an active and trusted resource behind the social media profile. Letting followers see that there is a reaction from a healthcare professional, no matter whether engaging with an advocate or antagonist, implies a caring expert is at the keyboard. Most importantly, asking the detractor to email or call directly can keep social media comments from escalating. Often, detractors will not follow-up at all. If they do, the situation should be addressed by a patient relations team, manager, or another individual who is trained to engage with complainants. Apologies to the detractor are not recommended, as they can imply fault and be used in future litigation. No matter what the complaint protocol is, it is important to stick to it and address all detractors with consistent language and tone.

Crisis Communication

One of the worst scenarios a healthcare professional can imagine is a large-scale, catastrophic event that includes mass numbers of wounded who need care. Unfortunately, this occurrence is not as unusual as it may seem. When the public is looking for information, updates, and news surrounding the event, they turn to social media and any healthcare professional affiliated with the facility that is providing this critical care. A good start to communicating updates is to have a template that addresses initial inquiries. It might look something like this:

We are currently responding to _____. Updates will be posted on [insert web address] as soon as they become available. Families concerned for loved ones can gather at _____ or call _____.

A crisis communication template assures consistent, clear, and concise messages being posted organization-wide. This helps prevent overtly emotional status updates and the sharing of misinformation. Unless approved to do so by their organization, healthcare professionals should never talk to news media during a crisis, nor should

Fig. 9.4 Social media best
practices include not
posting pictures during a
crisis. (Adapted from
https://twitter.com/
JonnyM421)

Jonathan Moore
@JonnyM421

Follow

Sunrise Hospital, Las Vegas. Not a war zone.

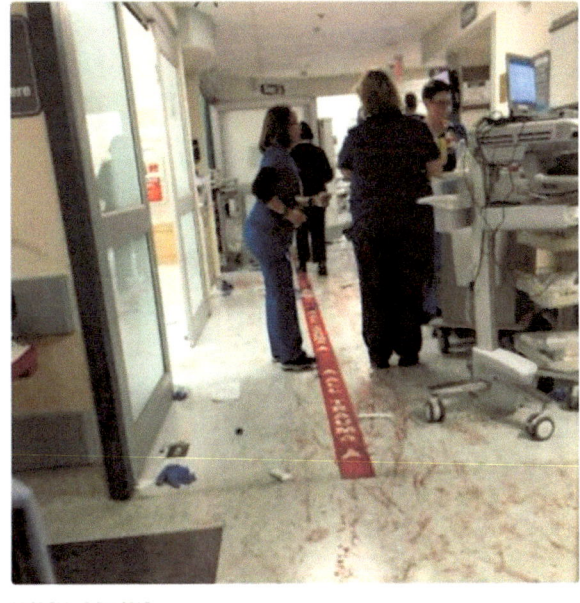

12:20 PM - 2 Oct 2017

888 Retweets 1,440 Likes

they share or retweet social media content for the same reasons. A media update is
only as good as its source and in the time of a crisis when reporters are trying to be
the first and fastest to break a story, there is not always a great deal of care being
taken to prevent falsities. As always, care should be taken to prevent the sharing of
PHI, so it is a best practice to never share pictures during a crisis, Fig. 9.4.

Maintain Appropriate Professional Boundaries

Social media can be a great venue in which to offer general health and wellness
information and best practices. Being a trusted resource to whom consumers and
peers can turn to is the true hallmark of healthcare social media. However, given the
opportunity, conversations can easily delve into a less-professional state. Boundaries
can be blurred when forums move outside of an exam room and onto a social media
feed. In order to maintain respectable distance, healthcare professionals should
never friend, follow, or fan a page or profile owned by, or run by, a patient or their
family. While it is common practice for patients and families to follow physicians

and healthcare organizations on social media for their knowledge and expertise, proper boundaries must be maintained at all times. Social media gives healthcare professionals a unique opportunity to provide accurate, evidence-based resources and information, but specific treatment or advice is poor practice. This does not have to result in a barrier to care; users can always be told to contact their physician or schedule an appointment.

Organizational Reputation

Whether it is being used to increase revenue, obtain speaking engagements, drive referrals or as brand advocacy, a well-run social media account can be instrumental in creating a community. An individual who is a known affiliate of an organization is a representative of that brand to their community, whether or not they disclose it in their social media profiles. This includes what they post on social media and what other users may post about them. The social media policy should instill awareness about how peers and consumers are currently using online platforms in order to help keep reputations intact. Social media for healthcare professionals is not always about what someone posts but how they treat their patients, co-workers, neighbors, and every person with whom they come in contact. A disgruntled patient family can post a dissatisfactory comment about a healthcare worker on Twitter or Facebook in a matter of seconds. Understanding that individual actions can reflect upon an organization's reputation is key to social media success.

Conclusion

Medical professionals and healthcare organizations should develop and/or adhere to guidelines that ensure best practices are always followed on social media. While this may seem like a deterrent for some professionals to engage on social media, this can serve as a useful tool to help guide online presence. Patient privacy must always be protected, and medical professionals are best served to avoid any potential controversy. With practice and time, any medical professional can develop an online reputation and safely engage with a wide audience.

References

1. Office for Civil Rights. Health information privacy. 6 Nov 2015. Retrieved 17 Sept 2018 from Health and Human Services. https://www.hhs.gov/hipaa/for-professionals/privacy/special-topics/de-identification/index.html#standard.
2. Office for Civil Rights. Guidance regarding methods for de-identification of protected health information in accordance with the health insurance portability and accountability act (HIPAA) privacy rule. 6 Nov 2015. Retrieved 17 Sept 2018 from Health and Human Services. https://www.hhs.gov/hipaa/for-professionals/privacy/special-topics/de-identification/index.html.

3. Smith A, Anderson M. Social media use in 2018. 1 Mar 2018. Retrieved 10 Aug 2018 from Pew Internet. http://www.pewinternet.org/2018/03/01/social-media-use-in-2018/.
4. United States Copyright Office. Subject matter and scope of copyright. Retrieved 29 Sept 2018 from Copyright.gov. https://www.copyright.gov/title17/92chap1.html#107.
5. The growing commons. Retrieved 2 Dec 2018 from Creative Commons. https://creativecommons.org/.
6. Creative Commons licenses. Retrieved 30 Sept 2018 from Creative Commons. https://creativecommons.org/licenses/.
7. Raychale. The 8 best ways to increase social media engagement for your brand. 17 Mar 2018. Retrieved 2 Dec 2018 from Lyfe Marketing. https://www.lyfemarketing.com/blog/increase-social-media-engagement/.
8. McCausland P, Melber A, Marinaccio D. Analysis: does Obama have grounds to sue Trump for libel? 6 Mar 2017. Retrieved 29 Sept 2018 from NBC News. https://www.nbcnews.com/news/us-news/analysis-does-obama-have-grounds-sue-trump-libel-n729376.
9. Defamation. Retrieved 20 Sept 2018 from Cornell Law School's Legal Information Institute. https://www.law.cornell.edu/wex/defamation.
10. Weaver J. 16 July 2018. Retrieved from 29 Sept 2018 from NBC News. http://www.nbcnews.com/id/3077086/t/more-people-search-health-online/#.XASOXotKiM8.
11. Cooper T, Allen S. 2018 global health care outlook. 2018. Retrieved from Deloitte. https://www2.deloitte.com/global/en/pages/life-sciences-and-healthcare/articles/global-health-care-sector-outlook.html.

How to Spot and Deal with Internet Trolls

10

Callista M. Dammann

Most people, when they think of an insult, they keep it to themselves. But you wouldn't believe the things people say on my Twitter feed, and I'm a nice guy. Imagine if I was a jerk.

—Jeff Ross, The RoastMaster General

How to Deal with Trolls: Strategies for Dealing with Negative Comments and Feedback

Like death and taxes, an inevitability of gaining notoriety in the social media realm is dealing with trolls. No, we're not talking about gemstone-bellied forest creatures voiced by Justin Timberlake (but those would be far more pleasant); we're talking about social media trolls.

A troll is a person who posts irrelevant, inflammatory, or offensive content online meant to disrupt a conversation or provoke or upset others. "Trolling" is simply the act of posting this type of content. The main goal of almost all trolls is to create conflict. In the case of medical professionals, it is often a social media troll's goal to create distrust in an individual's practices or the medical community as a whole.

It is important to note that disagreeing with someone on the Internet does not constitute trolling. The Internet is full of disagreements or conversations offering differing viewpoints. This type of conflict and conversation should be expected when sparking a discussion or debate online. Unfortunately, there will be few topics where the whole of the Internet, or even your followers, will agree with you 100 percent. Even when you are sharing your own peer-reviewed research findings, do not expect everyone to be in your camp of thought. But once again, this is simply debate and not trolling.

So, how do you spot a social media troll versus someone who simply disagrees with you? Well, in most cases, it's actually pretty easy. Let's start by looking at the facts when it comes to trolling.

© Springer Nature Switzerland AG 2019
D. R. Stukus et al., *Social Media for Medical Professionals*,
https://doi.org/10.1007/978-3-030-14439-5_10

A 2016 Online Harassment Study showed that 25% of American adults report being bullied or harassed online [1]. A 2014 study by Pew Research Center found that 73% of adult Internet users have seen someone being harassed in some way online [2]. Since many trolling behaviors fall into the harassment category, while you may not have been personally trolled, statistics show that it is highly likely you have seen this type of behavior on social media.

Trolls have varying extremes of conversation disruption and are often categorized by the types of behavior or responses they convey. Like all topics on the Internet, there is no consistent way to classify trolls (in fact we've seen lists with as few as 4 types of trolls and as many as 100), so for the sake of this book, here are the six most common troll types we have seen interact with healthcare professionals and how we suggest dealing with them. We'll start with the easy ones!

Types of Trolls

The Grammar and Spelling Troll

You send a tweet with the incorrect form of "there/their/they're." In your haste of typing a Facebook post on your iPhone's keyboard, you miss an apostrophe. Think no one will notice? The grammar and spelling troll will, and they'll sometimes throw in a little insult about your character or education when correcting you. Their commentary is often passive-aggressive and annoying, but in reality, they are a fairly easy troll to deal with. If the spelling or grammar mistake they pointed out is on a channel where you have the ability to edit your post, correct it and thank the troll for pointing out your mistake. If you can't correct it (i.e., Twitter), you can still send out a quick, "Thanks for letting me know!" Overall, taking the high ground and being pleasant with this troll will typically make your life easier. If they continue to comment on your post, adding in some insults or harsh language, we suggest simply ignoring them. They'll go away once the conversation becomes one-sided.

If you want to avoid the grammar and spelling troll altogether, we suggest following the age-old advice "read three times, post once." You may still make a mistake here and there, after all, we're only human, but odds are, you will catch a lot of your mistakes before they are even posted.

The Political Troll

The political troll likes to attack any and all political messaging that isn't from their political party. In many cases their attack has nothing to do with the issue itself, but rather the fact that your side of the issue does not fall within their party lines. Why do we mention this troll, you ask? It may seem strange considering politics are not your profession; however healthcare is a big part of the political scene. If you are a part of a healthcare organization or hospital, they may ask you to share a statement or messaging advocating on behalf of your patient population when it comes to

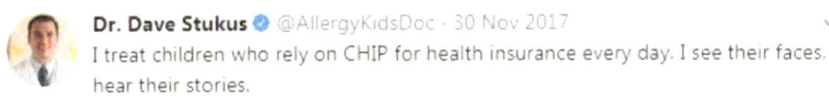

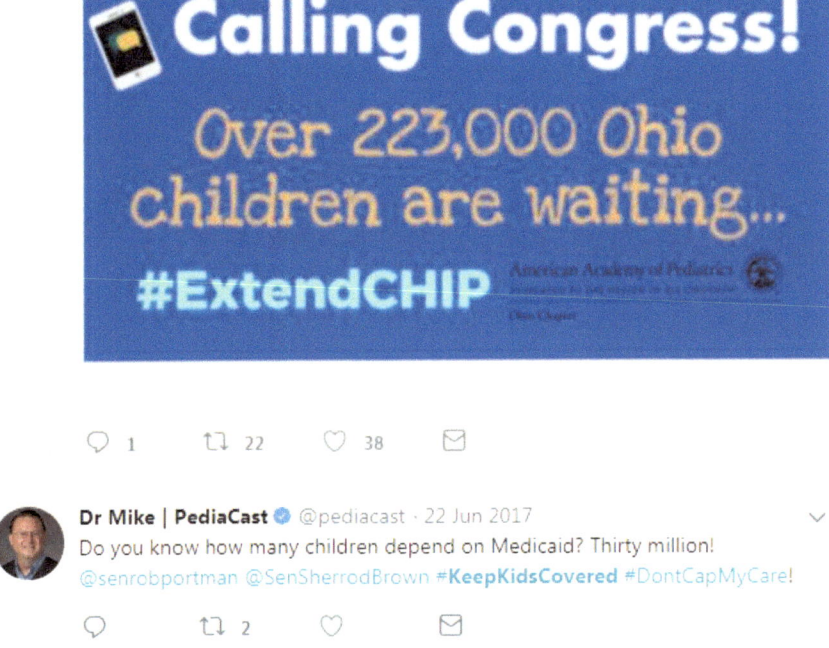

Fig. 10.1 Examples of tweets shared by physicians related to political issues that affect health-care. This type of political post can often draw the attention of political trolls. (Adapted from https://twitter.com/AllergyKidsDoc)

certain political issues. If the issue is something you believe in and support, it is absolutely okay for you to share this messaging on your social media channels; we encourage it! Just be prepared for the trolls. In Fig. 10.1, you can see a Medicare tweet co-author, Dr. Mike Patrick, shared on Twitter as well as a tweet related to CHIP funding shared by co-author, Dr. David Stukus. Luckily, neither of them had any trolling attacks related to these particular messages, but you always need to be prepared when talking politics!

If you are sharing messaging about a Democrat-backed policy, expect attacks from Republican political trolls. Vice versa, if you are sharing messaging from a Republican-backed policy, expect Democrat political trolls to come out swinging! Regardless of party, the political troll often does not attack the issue itself but instead uses social media to attack your perceived alliance to the political party that is not their own. They may also attack based on who they think you voted for in a particular election race, or they may attack the patient population the issue affects. In the case of the political troll, it is best to ignore them. It is unlikely your tweet or Facebook comment is going to persuade them to change their political views.

The Insult Troll

The insult troll is someone who will insult anyone and everyone for absolutely no reason. They are true cyberbullies, engaging in any tactic that will get a person riled up. From name-calling to unfounded accusations, their "mean girl" persona can be seen in any and all interactions they have on social media. How should you deal with this type of troll? Avoid responding to them at all costs. No good will come from engaging with this person. If they do persist in engaging with your posts or tweets, considering reporting their account or blocking them. It will make your life easier in the end.

The Bad Experience Troll

The bad experience troll is just that – someone who had a real or perceived bad experience with you or your practice. Now, please know that voicing their concerns about their experience does not make them a troll. If they share their concern on social media, respond to them, but take the conversation offline. Let them know you hear them, and provide them with a phone number to call or ask that they come to your office so you can discuss the experience over the phone or face to face. A standard response could be, "Hi [name]. Thank you for reaching out. I would like to talk with you more about your experience. Please call/email [provide contact information]." If your hospital or practice has a patient relations department, talk with them about the best way to handle complaints on social media. They may suggest triaging all complaints through their department.

As discussed many times throughout this book, it is important to remind healthcare professionals that you should never share patient information online. If the person sharing the complaint asks why they cannot discuss their experience online, let them know it is against HIPAA policies.

So what makes someone go from a person who wants to make a complaint to a bad experience troll? In our experience, it is that the issue does not get resolved. If a person sees you as ignoring their concerns or the follow-up to a concern is not to their satisfaction, this is when you may see the bad experience troll come out. From your Twitter and Facebook posts to reviews about you and your practice on Google, Vitals, or Healthgrades, this troll finds every place they can to complain about their experience and drag your name and reputation through the mud. How do you deal with this troll? Well if you have not already talked to them in person or over the phone about their experience, do so! Sometimes the simple act of reaching out makes a person feel heard and validated, and they will stop posting. If you've already reached out and spoken to the person once, reach out a second time. There may be something they feel you could have or should have done after your initial follow-up that will help you to rectify the situation.

In some extreme cases, no matter how many times you speak with them, the bad experience troll will not go away. They may continue to post the same story over and over in the comments section of your posts. They may put a 1-star review of you on every site they can find. If you truly feel you have done everything in your power to rectify the situation and they continue to troll your accounts, we suggest reporting their account to the social media platform and/or blocking them from your account where possible. If the information shared in their reviews is true, make sure you do not remove it. This could make things even worse. However, if it is untrue, you can report their individual review to whatever site it is on and ask that it be removed. It is unlikely you will run into a situation this extreme, but it has happened before and we want you to be prepared.

The Topic Trolls (Also Known as the Persistent Debate Troll)

The topic troll, like the bad experience troll, can be incredibly difficult to deal with. This is the troll we most often see attacking healthcare professionals, so it is important to understand them. When it comes to topic trolls, it is often not just one individual who attacks you but a whole group of people. This group of people has banded together to fight for or against one particular topic. In healthcare, we've seen this type of trolling to be most prevalent when discussing vaccinations and circumcision, but there are a whole slew of healthcare-related topics that this type of troll attacks.

So how does the topic troll come to light? Let's walk through an example. As a healthcare professional, you may have decided to share a tweet about why it is important to get your flu shot, such as the tweet sent by co-author, Dr. David Stukus, Fig. 10.2.

Unfortunately for Dr. Stukus, there is a whole group of people on Twitter who are strongly against the flu shot. Their minds are not going to be changed on this topic, and they look for every chance to state their viewpoint. Some topic trolls have an arsenal of articles they point to every time they see a pro flu shot tweet. Some look at every tweet individually and try to dissect it in a way to prove the person's message wrong. In the case of Dr. Stukus' tweet above, several people looked at fact number three and said "Wait, 20% got the flu shot and died?" and then went on in various ways to question the effectiveness of the vaccine.

When it comes to topic trolls, sometimes the responses will appear on your social media post for a few hours, sometimes days, sometimes weeks. So, how do you respond? In truth you have two options. One – and always our best advice – ignore

Dr. Dave Stukus ✔
@AllergyKidsDoc

Follow

Here are 3 indisputable #facts:
1. It is 2018.
2. 172 children in the United States died from influenza this winter season.
3. 80% of them did not receive the #flushot.

This virus does not care about your beliefs. It kills children. Every. Single. Year.

Pittsburgh Post-Gazette ✔ @PittsburghPG
The worst flu season in recent years is over bit.ly/2HD9viv

4:45 PM · 11 Jun 2018

Fig. 10.2 A tweet sent by Dr. David Stukus about the importance of getting your annual flu shot. (Adapted from https://twitter.com/AllergyKidsDoc)

the troll or group of trolls entirely. You are not going to change their mind with your post, tweet, or an article you share.

If you do feel compelled to respond, wait. Sit on your response for 12–24 hours. In the social media world, that likely seems like a long time. And it is. But we are human; waiting will give you time to gather your thoughts and to respond from a place of thoughtfulness and articulation rather than a place of exhaustion and anger.

Figure 10.3 is a great example of how you can use your response to educate your followers as a whole. Dr. Stukus is responding to a topic troll who claims flu vaccines do not work because they are inactivated. By using quote tweet in the response, he is showing his followers both the myth and the facts related to flu vaccines.

If you do decide to respond to a topic troll as Dr. Stukus did, be prepared for more trolls. Sometimes they do not respond, but oftentimes responding just makes them attack more, and they may bring their social media "friends" into the mix to attack you as well.

If you are passionate about an issue that a group of people are passionate against, there is no avoiding the topic troll. What you can do is choose to be thoughtful and articulate each time you post about the topic on your social media channel. Reread your words multiple times before posting, and if you have the time, look for ways

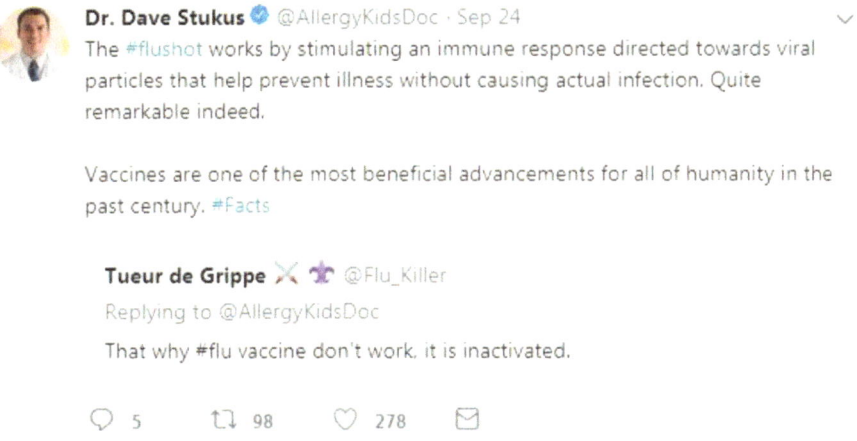

Fig. 10.3 An example of a way to respond to topic trolls. Utilizing the quote tweet functionality of Twitter, Dr. Stukus has used a topic troll's tweet to dispel a myth about the flu vaccine for his followers. (Adapted from https://twitter.com/AllergyKidsDoc)

that someone may be able to pick it apart before posting. You may find you already have a great response to an argument against what you are sharing. Make sure that your post has facts and statistics to support it. Prepare yourself for the trolls, but know that there is likely nothing you can say to change their minds.

Extremist Troll

It is incredibly rare that you would interact with an extremist troll, but we want to mention them in the book because they do exist. The extremist troll is not just a troll; they take their trolling and negative behaviors to the next level.

So what makes an extremist troll? This is someone who goes beyond negative comments and makes physical threats against you or family members, contacts your employer with false claims about you or your practice, and/or creates a website or social media account dedicated to their extreme dislike of you. This and similar behaviors can and should be reported.

1. Report their account to the social media platform. According to the Online Harassment Study [1] we discussed earlier, 61% of accounts reported for harassment were shut down by the social media network.
2. Let your employer know if you are being attacked by this type of troll. As stated before, they will often contact your employer with false claims about you. Your employer may have additional steps they would like you to take.
3. If you feel threatened, contact local law enforcement.

Online harassment is a crime, and the extremist troll is not someone you should have to deal with on your own.

Tips for Dealing with Trolls

We discussed strategies for dealing with the six most common troll types, but in reality there are even more trolls out there and new types of trolls being created each day. If you come across a troll we did not discuss, here is our best advice for dealing with them.

The number one way to deal with any troll: Ignore them. Completely. Let's revisit the Pew Internet Research Survey [2] we discussed earlier. When it comes to online harassment, 60% of respondents said they simply chose to ignore the person entirely. Most often when dealing with a troll, this is the best course of action. By ignoring them, you are not giving them more information to react and respond to. Many trolls argue for arguments sake. You may continue to see them respond to your posts, making rude and unnecessary commentary, but even if they do this, the vast number of trolls will simply go away when you ignore their comments.

Choosing not to respond to a troll can be difficult. So if you are going to respond, make sure your argument is well thought out. As we mentioned before, wait 12–24 hours before responding to your trolls. This may seem like a long time in the social media world – and it is. But as humans, we need the time to calm down and think of truly thoughtful and articulate responses. Often responding right away has us responding from our hearts and not our brains. It's easy to lash out at someone, especially when they are trying to prove your profession or your research wrong. Taking the time to allow yourself to be in their shoes and see where they are coming from can allow you to provide a thoughtful, evidence-based response. You will often find that they still disagree with you – after all that's the root of what a troll is there to do – but at least you don't come across as being a troll yourself.

What if the trolling gets truly out of hand? Well you have a few options:

1. You can block or unfriend the person.
2. You can report the account to the platform they are trolling you on. Each platform has a unique reporting process but the "report" button is always clearly displayed within the tweet/comments.
3. Turn off commenting. This is only possible if you are utilizing a platform such as Facebook, Instagram, or a personal blog where you have the ability to take this action.

Last but not least: **Don't feed the trolls**.

Unfortunately there are some topics that inevitably lend themselves to trolling. In training physicians on the do's and don'ts of social media, we often ask the question, "What healthcare topics do you think get the most attention from trolls on social media?" The first two answers we always receive are vaccinations and circumcision. Both of these topics have a strong community both for and against their practice; therefore, the mention of either topic will bring out a community of attackers. Depending on the information you share, you may find that your post either becomes the subject of a lively and heated debate for a few hours or a few days – or you may find yourself with your very own set of social media trolls. Either way, you need to be prepared to hear from them, and more importantly, you need to be prepared to ignore them. Responding to trolls is almost always a bad idea, and every minute you spend getting worked up about what they have to say is a minute you aren't spending with your family, your friends, and your patients. In summary, it's simply not worth it to spend your time worrying about trolls.

So, Why Do People Become Social Media Trolls? (And How Not to Turn into One)

Why do people become social media trolls? There are many reasons why people may become trolls, but let's look at the four biggest reasons.

1. *Anonymity*. If you look at many of the trolls who gain notoriety on social media, they go by a pseudonym, and they do not have a photo of themselves associated with their account. In short, they can be anonymous. Even for those that do have a real name and photo associated with their account, there is still a certain degree of anonymity. Why? You aren't talking to a person face to face. You are likely not even talking to someone in your own hometown. More than half of the comments you read online, you probably think, "I can't believe someone would say that!" And in truth, they never would if this were an in-person discussion or debate. Sitting behind a computer screen and keyboard somehow make people bolder. They say far more than they ever would in a real-life discussion.
2. *Herd mentality*. The beauty of the Internet is that you can find a lot of people just like you! It's the downfall of the Internet as well. If you only surround yourself with people who have the same views and opinions that you have, it's easy to see the other side as inherently "wrong." Let's go back to the flu vaccine example we gave earlier. If you are against the flu vaccine and surround yourself with followers who are also against the flu vaccine, it's easy to jump on the bandwagon with them and attack anyone who feels differently.
3. *Personality*. Some people are just inherently more prone to becoming social media trolls than others. Do you know someone who enjoys getting others riled up? Someone who is inherently outspoken? What about someone who sees themselves as better than others? All of these traits and many others can make a person more susceptible to becoming a social media troll.
4. *Everybody else is doing it*. Think about it. How frequently do you see comments from social media trolls? Weekly? Daily? Hourly? We see them so frequently; we've become desensitized to the comments. That level of desensitization makes

it easier for us to post the negative comments that come to our own minds. You may start by just posting one negative comment thinking, what's the harm? There are so many others. But that could send you down the spiral of becoming a troll yourself.

As you can see, there are a lot of reasons why a person may become a social media troll stemming from their own personality traits to the types of commentary we expose ourselves to regularly online. So, how can you get involved in social media without becoming a troll yourself? Try not to get bogged down by the negativity of social media. Understand that not everyone is going to have the same opinion that you do. Even if you cannot see their side of the argument, do not attack a person because their beliefs differ from your own. Use your social media platforms to spread the messages you want to get across to your follower – your family, friends, and patients – don't use them to attack the other side. Be the better person in arguments and debates. And take your mom's advice; "If you don't have anything nice to say, don't say anything at all."

How to Have a Healthy and Productive Debate Online

Now that we have taken a deeper dive into trolling, let's take a few minutes to talk about how to be involved in a healthy and productive debate online. The first thing to note is that when it comes to healthcare, people are going to have differing opinions. In fact, oftentimes people truthfully want to have an open and honest dialogue about a topic, especially when it concerns their or a family member's health. As you begin your trek into sharing information on a social media platform, most experts would suggest sharing research studies or facts related to areas of medicine that you specialize in or that interest you. For example, an allergist may want to share the latest peanut allergy study, and a gastroenterologist may want to share the latest breakthroughs in treating Crohn's disease. Sharing this type of evidence-based information is definitely the right way to start you on your path to being a go-to expert in your field on social media.

One co-author of this book, Dr. David Stukus, regularly has productive debates through his Twitter account on "Myth Buster Monday." During this time, he focuses on some of the myths he has heard within his practice, on social media, or in the news and shares the facts along with additional evidence-based resources to back up his point when needed. Figure 10.4 offers a few examples:

A myth is a widely held but false belief. So in sharing this information, Dr. Stukus knows there are plenty of people out there who disagree with him. So why share this information? Doesn't it go against the advice we've been giving this entire chapter of "Don't feed the trolls"? Not necessarily.

When sharing these myths, Dr. Stukus not only shares the truth about a particular myth; he also backs this up with evidence-based research, a peer-reviewed article, or a blog post from a credible medical person or institution.

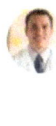

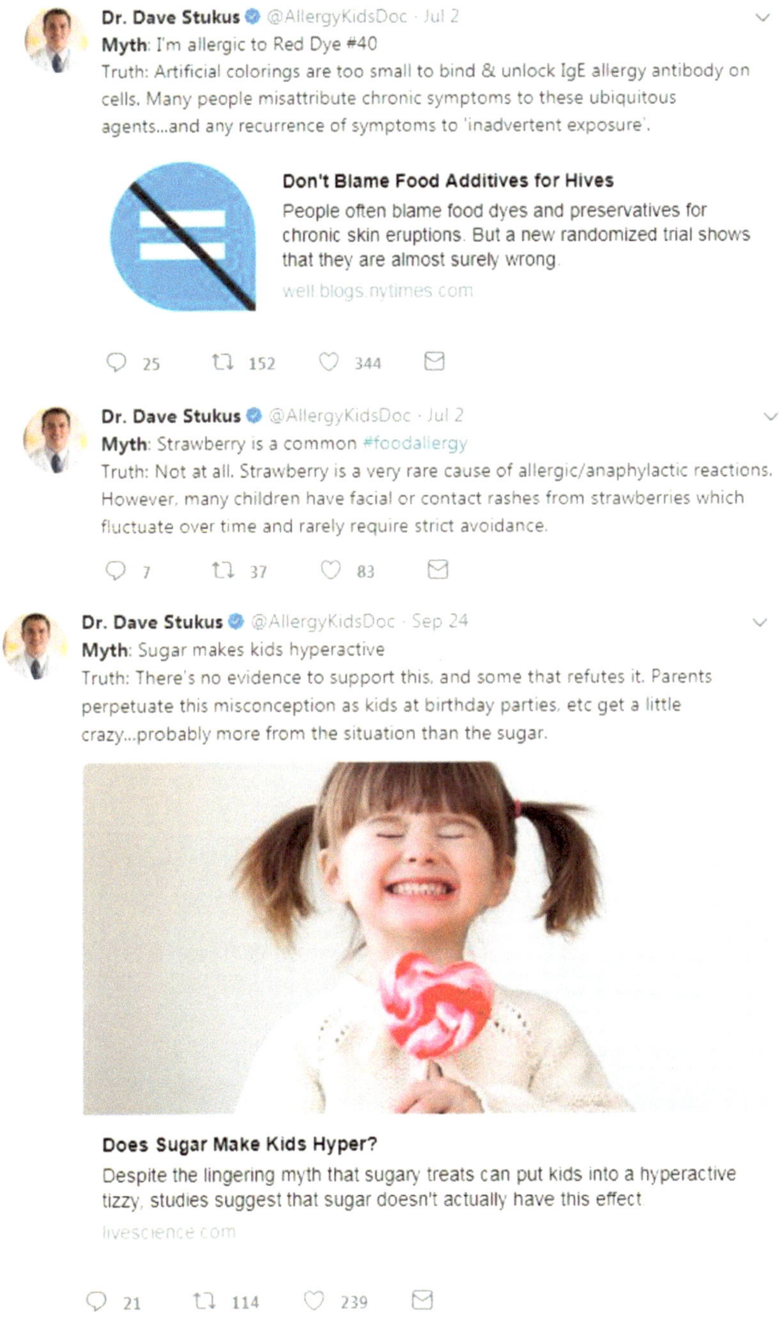

Dr. Dave Stukus ✔ @AllergyKidsDoc · Jul 2

Myth: I'm allergic to Red Dye #40

Truth: Artificial colorings are too small to bind & unlock IgE allergy antibody on cells. Many people misattribute chronic symptoms to these ubiquitous agents...and any recurrence of symptoms to 'inadvertent exposure'.

Don't Blame Food Additives for Hives

People often blame food dyes and preservatives for chronic skin eruptions. But a new randomized trial shows that they are almost surely wrong.

well.blogs.nytimes.com

◯ 25   �recycle 152   ♡ 344   ✉

Dr. Dave Stukus ✔ @AllergyKidsDoc · Jul 2

Myth: Strawberry is a common #foodallergy

Truth: Not at all. Strawberry is a very rare cause of allergic/anaphylactic reactions. However, many children have facial or contact rashes from strawberries which fluctuate over time and rarely require strict avoidance.

◯ 7   �recycle 37   ♡ 83   ✉

Dr. Dave Stukus ✔ @AllergyKidsDoc · Sep 24

Myth: Sugar makes kids hyperactive

Truth: There's no evidence to support this, and some that refutes it. Parents perpetuate this misconception as kids at birthday parties, etc get a little crazy...probably more from the situation than the sugar.

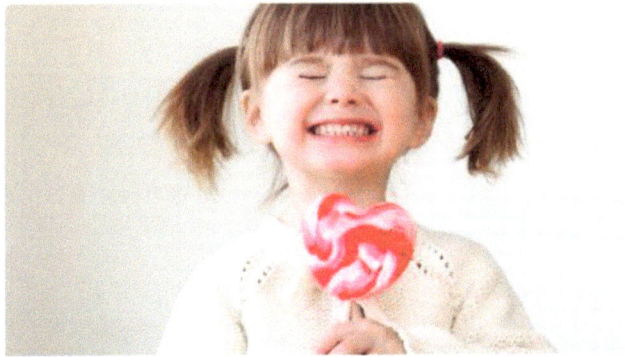

Does Sugar Make Kids Hyper?

Despite the lingering myth that sugary treats can put kids into a hyperactive tizzy, studies suggest that sugar doesn't actually have this effect.

livescience.com

◯ 21   �recycle 114   ♡ 239   ✉

Fig. 10.4 A few examples of "Myth Buster Monday" tweets shared by Dr. David Stukus. These tweets often spark a productive debate or conversation from both patients and colleagues. (Adapted from https://twitter.com/AllergyKidsDoc)

Also, he does not attribute them to a single person or group of people. By not including the person or group of people who believe the myth or misinformation, he is able to be perceived positively, as someone giving general medical advice on social media.

Finally, when Dr. Stukus receives questions regarding his myth buster tweets, he responds thoughtfully and articulately. Since each of these is a common misconception, there are a lot of people with questions when he sends out this type of tweet. Figure 10.5 depicts an example of a great interaction between him and another Twitter account related to teens and medication. It does not appear that he changes the users mind, but both sides clearly articulate their side of the argument and no unnecessary trolling ensues!

As we mentioned at the beginning of this chapter, social media debates are not necessarily trolling. However, if you find a lively debate going in the direction of trolling, stop responding. You are not going to change their minds, and it is not worth your time to continue to respond.

Dr. Dave Stukus ✓
@AllergyKidsDoc

Following ⌄

Myth: My teen should be responsible for their own medicine
Truth: Even if they want to, they likely can't be. Normal cognitive development during adolescence involves a lack of appreciating long term consequences. Parental supervision & reminder systems can improve nonadherence.

6:30 PM · 2 Jul 2018

88 Retweets 307 Likes

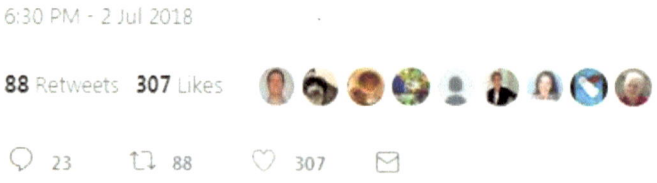

♡ 23   ⟲ 88   ♡ 307   ✉

Fig. 10.5 An example of a productive conversation on one of Dr. Stukus' Myth Buster Monday tweets. It's easy to have productive conversations and debates online when you are thoughtful and articulate in your conversation. (Adapted from https://twitter.com/AllergyKidsDoc)

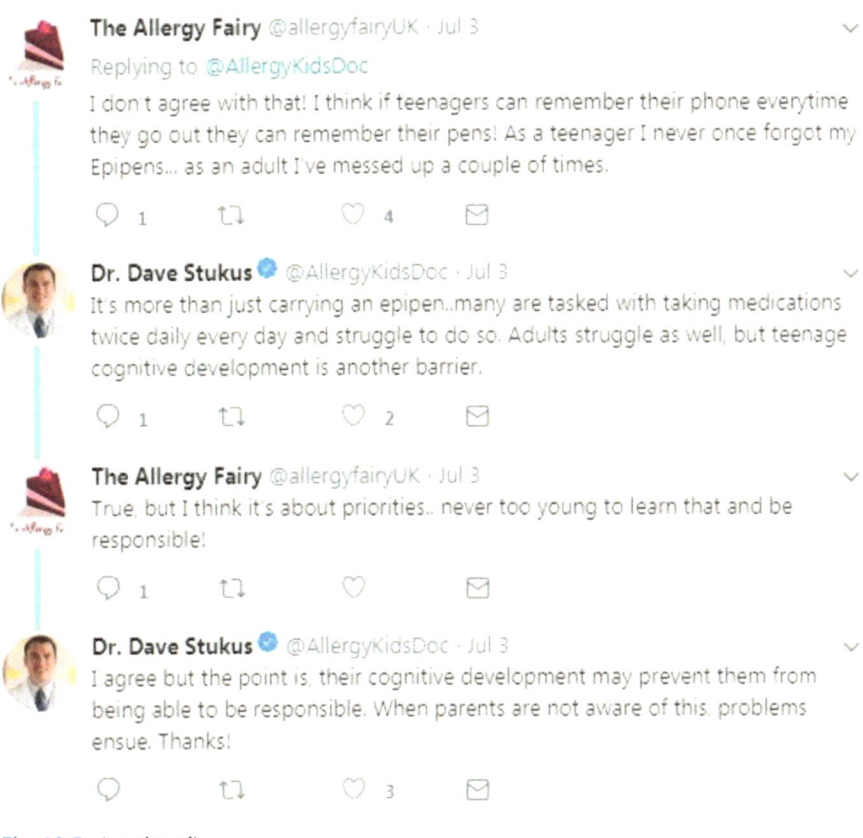

The Allergy Fairy @allergyfairyUK · Jul 3

Replying to @AllergyKidsDoc

I don't agree with that! I think if teenagers can remember their phone everytime they go out they can remember their pens! As a teenager I never once forgot my Epipens... as an adult I've messed up a couple of times.

♡ 1   ⇄   ♡ 4   ✉

Dr. Dave Stukus ✓ @AllergyKidsDoc · Jul 3

It's more than just carrying an epipen..many are tasked with taking medications twice daily every day and struggle to do so. Adults struggle as well, but teenage cognitive development is another barrier.

♡ 1   ⇄   ♡ 2   ✉

The Allergy Fairy @allergyfairyUK · Jul 3

True, but I think it's about priorities.. never too young to learn that and be responsible!

♡ 1   ⇄   ♡   ✉

Dr. Dave Stukus ✓ @AllergyKidsDoc · Jul 3

I agree but the point is, their cognitive development may prevent them from being able to be responsible. When parents are not aware of this, problems ensue. Thanks!

♡   ⇄   ♡ 3   ✉

Fig. 10.5 (continued)

Conclusion

As you begin to gain a following on social media, know that attracting a troll or two is inevitable. Do not let the fear of attracting them stop you from sharing your message. Continue to share the facts about medicine and healthcare through evidence-based studies and peer-reviewed articles. In almost all cases, choosing not to respond is the best way to deal with trolls, but if you do feel compelled to respond, be thoughtful and articulate in everything you post. Resist the urge to utilize troll tactics in your responses like bullying and name-calling. Be the better person. And when all else fails, follow these two rules:

1. **Don't feed the trolls!**
2. Remember mom's advice from your grade school days, "If you don't have anything nice to say, don't say anything at all!"

References

1. Rad Campaign, Lincoln Park Strategies, Craig Connects. The rise of online harassment. In: The rise of online harassment; 2016. http://www.onlineharassmentdata.org/. Accessed 10 Sep 2018.
2. Duggan M. Online harassment | Pew Research Center. In: Pew Research Center: Internet, Science & Tech; 2015. http://www.pewinternet.org/2014/10/22/online-harassment/. Accessed 10 Sept 2018.

The Sky Is the Limit

11

David R. Stukus

> *It isn't enough to think outside the box. Thinking is passive. Get used to acting outside the box.*
>
> —Tim Ferriss

Social Media and the Ivory Tower

Traditionally, academic institutions have used time-honored metrics to determine promotion and tenure for faculty members. In general, academic accomplishments are considered in realms such as clinical practice, research, and education [1]. The number of peer-reviewed publications, invited editorials, and book chapters written by a faculty member demonstrate how they have contributed to the acquisition and dissemination of knowledge. The little discussed paradox of this approach is the inherent limitation in dissemination of information through publishing one's original work in peer-reviewed medical journals. Many journals have hefty subscription fees and individual articles, and although indexed publicly on sites such as PubMed or Google Scholar, cannot be accessed without payment. It is also impossible for any medical professional to keep up with the volumes of new research and scientific discovery taking place every year. Even the most dedicated academician must choose how they will discover new publications relevant to their interests and then find time to read and interpret each article. All of these factors limit the actual number of people who will ever read someone's peer-reviewed publication (especially from beginning to end).

However, as demonstrated throughout this textbook, social media allows for a very different and wider reaching platform where any medical professional can grow an audience and disseminate their information. While most peer-reviewed publications may lie behind pay walls, medical professionals can still contribute original ideas and educate others by sharing their comments, opinions, blog posts, tweets, infographics, YouTube videos, or Facebook posts. Traditionally, the impact

© Springer Nature Switzerland AG 2019
D. R. Stukus et al., *Social Media for Medical Professionals*,
https://doi.org/10.1007/978-3-030-14439-5_11

of peer-reviewed publications has been measured by number of citations in other publications. The more times someone's work is cited by others, the more this demonstrates the importance, impact, and relevance of their work. However, it takes years to build citations. By the time a researcher develops a hypothesis for testing, obtains funding for their original research idea, conducts their study, interprets the data, writes and edits their manuscript, submits their manuscript, awaits peer-review and then additional edits (not to mention even more lags in time for papers that are rejected by journals and undergo several rounds of submission and peer-review), undergoes a time lag prior to publication, THEN must be discovered and read by others and await their own research timeline and manuscript preparation in order to be cited…this is a process that takes years, even decades. And that's just for one paper to accumulate citations. Thankfully, this has changed in recent years, and approaches such as altmetrics can use the entire Internet to better determine impact of an author's work by including citations not only in other peer-reviewed publications but also on Wikipedia, public policy documents, discussion forums on blog sites, media coverage, and mentions on social media. This approach has transformed how the impact of an author can be measured and assesses impact before the accrual of academic citations. Academic institutions have followed suit, and many have incorporated altmetrics into their criteria for promotion and tenure [2].

In 2016, the Mayo Clinic Academic Appointments and Promotions Committee began including digital and social media scholarship among criteria considered for academic achievement. Other institutions have followed suit and guidance for medical professionals seeking this path is available online [3] and through peer-reviewed publications [4, 5]. As discussed in earlier chapters, social media provides robust and specific data that users can gather and analyze. In lieu of waiting years to accumulate citations, a medical professional on social media can use metrics on Twitter or Facebook to immediately determine how many people have seen, clicked on, or interacted with their post. Altmetrics also allow users to capture how often their work is being disseminated or used by other online forums as well. Promotion and tenure committees often struggle with how to define, measure, and equalize the quality and impact of scholarly work among faculty candidates with differing backgrounds and scope of academic pursuits. Social media has the potential to help in this realm through use of metrics and a structured definition of scholarship [6].

Medical professionals who are interested in using their social media achievements in consideration for promotion should consult with their university's promotion and tenure guidelines and committee to see if guidelines already exist. This is an area that will evolve over time and likely have significant discrepancies between institutions. Some institutions may not value these contributions, whereas others may have clear guidelines on how to demonstrate the quality and reach of one's work. In general, it will be useful for medical professionals taking this pathway to promotion to demonstrate how they have used social media to complement their academic area of interest and expertise. It will not be good enough to submit a dossier and state "I have 5,000 Twitter followers" as a measure of one's impact. A clear description of one's philosophy in use of social media to augment scholarly activity will help those on the promotion and tenure committee who are unfamiliar with this approach. Additional description of one's audience as well as objectives and platforms used will be important as well. Lastly, a description of content creation, content curation, community management, data and metrics surrounding engagement, and a long-standing record of achievement will be imperative to demonstrate how and why social media should be considered as part of one's academic accomplishments.

In 2015, I was one of the first faculty members at my institution to attempt to use my social media involvement when I submitted my dossier for consideration of promotion from Assistant to Associate Professor of Pediatrics. I had a very productive discussion with the vice dean of academic affairs at my university who was not only supportive but helped me frame my "story" in a way that demonstrated my pioneering work in social media. Prior to our meeting, I viewed my work as a clinician, educator, and allergist as separate from my social media involvement. When evaluated separately and individually, each aspect was not robust or overly convincing. However, when I combined my achievements as a pediatric allergist/immunologist with my social media accomplishments, a more complete story was told. I also made sure I met the traditional criteria for teaching, clinical care, institutional service, research, and involvement in national organizations. In my dossier, I carefully characterized and provided data to support how my Twitter presence directly led to new patient referrals, invitations to present at national conferences, and national reputation as an allergist. My biggest challenge at the time was in conveying these social media accomplishments in the traditional language. Categorizing the number of publications, invited presentations, and involvement in national committees fell into the traditional checkboxes and certainly helped. At my institution, the promotion and tenure committee is comprised of physicians and faculty members with various backgrounds who are purposefully assigned dossiers to review for those outside their field. Thus, a tenured orthopedic surgeon with no knowledge of social media (or worse, a hatred of it!) could have been assigned my application, and I needed to demonstrate on paper how a pediatric allergist with a Twitter handle was worthy of promotion. In the end, I received my promotion, and there are now several examples of colleagues at my institution using their social media achievements to help with promotion. I promised myself that if I could pull that off, I would try to help anyone else I could. In 2016, I published a blog outlining my approach on the popular KevinMD site [3], and this textbook and chapter are part of my continued efforts to help others achieve their goals. Please feel free to message me on social media with questions…and especially with successful stories!

Public Health

Social media has been utilized to create global networks that can quickly spread information and mobilize large numbers of people to reach common goals related to public health [7]. State and local health departments use Twitter and other social media sites to help spread awareness and education to impact as many residents as possible [8]. Another unique and creative way public health departments and organizations use Twitter and social media is to track keyword content from other accounts. In combination with location tracking technology, this can assist the monitoring of population health [9]. For example, the Centers for Disease Control is very active on social media which is utilized to share updates and track conversations regarding infectious outbreaks across a population, such as influenza activity every autumn and winter. Other organizations such as the Red Cross have used Twitter to monitor posts during natural disasters and help determine where the greatest needs lie in real time. This two-way exchange of information highlights a remarkable manner in which social media can augment public health: by providing important health-related information to a wide population separated geographically and by socioeconomic status while also alerting organizations of any problems occurring among a similar diverse population in real time.

Given that social media is, after all, social, it can also be used as a way to influence public health behaviors. A unique example of this powerful impact occurred after Facebook allowed users to post their organ-donor status in their profile. The week after this feature was introduced, Donate Life America reported a 23-fold increase in donor pledges [7]! A systematic review published in 2014 identified 73 published articles/studies that evaluated the use of social media to influence public health [10]. Facebook was the most common single site (27%), and 34% of the studies utilized multiple sites. The range of topics in these studies was interesting, including attempts to reach individuals at risk for sexually transmitted diseases and connect them with available services, promotion of diabetes monitoring and management, and disease surveillance. Naturally, given their proclivity for using social media, adolescents and college students were the target audience for 44% of the studies in this review. Undoubtedly, the number of studies evaluating this approach to public health will increase in the coming years.

Research

The number of publications surrounding social media has increased markedly over the past 10 years and averages well more than a publication a day (Fig. 11.1). There are several themes surrounding the focus of these publications, including investigating how patients with specific medical conditions utilize social media, use of social media among medical professionals, how social media can be used for public health or patient education, and guidance for medical professionals surrounding social media best practices. In addition, these publications originate from multiple disciplines and specialties.

An interesting study published in 2018 looked through 1.5 million tweets to quantify and characterize which health conditions were being tweeted about most [11]. They found tweets related to 379 different health conditions, from over 450,000 Twitter users. There was a significant imbalance in size of communities and number of tweets for various health conditions, which informs us that medical professionals in some areas of specialty may have a wider audience

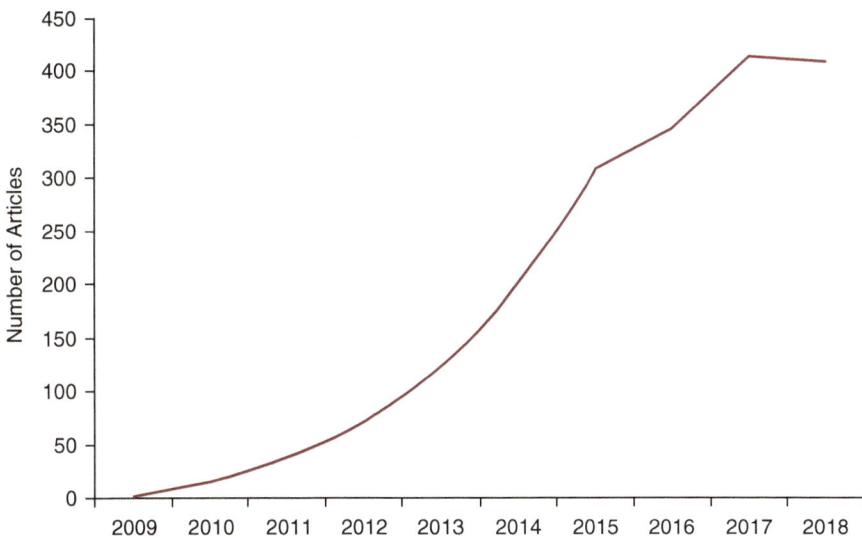

Fig. 11.1 Number of articles indexed in PubMed with search terms "Social Media Twitter"

on Twitter compared with others. In this study, autism, diabetes, dementia, AIDS, and post-traumatic stress disorder were the five most common health conditions according to total number of tweets. Rare conditions such as tuberous sclerosis, restenosis, stiff person syndrome, bone marrow failure, and Dupuytren's contracture had the fewest number of tweets. This type of analysis can be used over time, across various social media platforms, and even by geographic location to help medical professionals better understand how to find their target audience using social media.

As repeated throughout this textbook, a main reason that medical professionals should use social media is to combat the misinformation that patients and the public encounter online. Some clever research articles have investigated specific areas where social media has propagated non-evidence-based information. Let's revisit the attention grabbing 2014 Ebola outbreak that was initially introduced in Chap. 1. As discussed previously, this was the largest Ebola outbreak in history and was prominently reported on and discussed on social media channels. An editorial in the *British Medical Journal* published very shortly after the outbreak was initially contained commented on how information and misinformation on Twitter impacted the response from affected communities and healthcare responders [12]. One misguided recommendation that circulated (from nonmedical professionals) was through a hoax meme that urged Nigerians to drink excessive amounts of salt water to combat Ebola. While it is impossible to determine the direct effect of such tweets, media reports suggested this may have contributed to two deaths and more than a dozen hospitalizations.

Another unique study evaluated the depiction of asthma inhalers on Facebook, Twitter, and Instagram during two separate 3-day periods in 2016 [13]. Asthma is one of the most common chronic health conditions affecting both children and adults. Asthma inhalers are commonly used improperly due to incorrect technique, which leads to poor deposition of medication in the lower airways and reduced efficacy. Spacer devices are recommended to be used with metered dose inhalers to allow for aerosolization of the liquid medication and reduce deposition inside the mouth. The authors of this study identified 762 photos depicting inhaler use across all three platforms. Among these photos, correct inclusion of a spacer device was observed only 7.7% of the time. The authors conveyed concerns that patients with asthma seeking information online are likely to encounter incorrect depiction of inhaler technique, which may reinforce nonadherence and negatively impact their health outcomes. It will be interesting to see if similar future studies identify frequent incorrect technique on social media for other medical conditions requiring devices to deliver treatment, i.e., insulin injections for diabetes management or epinephrine injections for anaphylaxis.

Several research publications have investigated changes in the dynamic of the patient-provider relationship with the growth of social media. This is an important area for all of us to understand, regardless of which side of the relationship one falls on. A systematic review published in 2016 identified 22 studies that met their selection criteria [14]. Six categories of patient use of social media were identified: emotional, information, esteem, network support, social comparison, and emotional expression. These categories led to specific effects, including improved self-management, enhanced psychological well-being, social media addiction, and loss of privacy. The relationships between patients and medical professionals were affected in positive ways, including more equal communication between the patient and their provider and more harmonious relationships. Other consequences were observed as well, including increased switching of doctors (not always a bad thing) and suboptimal interaction between the patient and provider. Patients commented on reasons for joining online health communities, which included dissatisfaction with their healthcare professional's ability to meet their emotional and informational needs and to bridge the gap between health information from their provider and how to navigate everyday life with their medical condition. Another interesting reason was a belief that their medical professional was not aware of the latest breakthroughs, although it was not explored whether medical professionals with an online presence were deemed more up-to-date compared with their counterparts. We have discussed these gaps between patients and medical professionals previously, and data such as these are very informative and should be used to help the patient-provider relationship evolve in a productive and positive manner. While medical professionals may never (and likely should not) provide the emotional support patients may find through other patients in online support groups, they can anticipate reasons why their patients may seek information online and what types of interactions may deteriorate their relationship with them over time. Ideally, these discussions can take place in person before the relationship changes and may even strengthen these interactions. Hence, another example of how social media can help medical professionals provide anticipatory guidance to their patients in the clinical setting.

In Chap. 6, the use of Twitter at medical conferences was discussed as a way to increase user's engagement, enter into a wide ranging discussion, and increase visibility by using the conference hashtag during a time of focused engagement. There have been multiple publications surrounding the use of Twitter at medical conferences from various specialties, including, but not limited to, cardiology, allergy, surgical oncology, radiology, pathology, emergency medicine, urology, nephrology, and general surgery. Analysis of tweets using the hashtag #ESSO18 during a 2018 surgical oncology conference demonstrated 328 tweets from 58 users that generated more than seven million impressions during the 3-day conference [15]. That is not just free publicity for the organization and the specialty, but that represents millions of people receiving medical information being disseminated by a small number of users. While anyone can use a conference hashtag, including those not in attendance or potentially for misguided purposes, the majority of users are medical professionals who have established an online presence. Patients and the public view the information disseminated from medical conferences as cutting edge and from trusted sources. Longitudinal analysis has shown increased use of Twitter at annual meetings for Urology, Allergy, and Clinical Oncology conferences from across the world [16–18]. These data demonstrate that Twitter use from medical conferences is growing in popularity, is being adopted by multiple specialties, and is a worldwide phenomenon. Many meetings will not only advertise their official hashtag in the program and slide decks but also offer ribbons for participants to include on their name badges. This growing "club" of medical professionals who tweet from meetings is having a demonstrable and now measurable impact.

A randomized controlled trial (ideally, double blinded) is the gold standard methodology for research studies aiming to determine if one specific intervention results in a difference between two groups. Unfortunately, randomized trials are costly and time-consuming and require significant resources and support. In regard to social media, it is virtually impossible to conduct real-world randomized trials as participants would need to have all aspects of their online usage controlled to ensure blinding and prevent crossover. A clever study conducted by researchers at Haifa University in Israel utilized a controlled design with graduate students to examine the most effective way for health organizations to correct misinformation online surrounding measles vaccination [19]. In this study, 243 graduate students were randomized into two groups. Both groups were presented with the same dilemma of sending a child to kindergarten during a measles outbreak, knowing that some of the children in the school were not vaccinated due to their parents' objection. This was followed by an identical Facebook post shown to both groups voicing concerns from a mother of one of the kindergarten children that contained misinformation about measles and the ways it is contracted. In the third stage, the misinformation presented by the mother was corrected by an official health organization in two separate manners: one group received a brief unequivocal message containing facts about measles without any emotional element and the other group received information surrounding measles and how it is contracted, as well as reference to fears and concerns surrounding this situation, which was designed to communicate information transparently and address the public's concerns. The second group that received information transparently and with an element addressing emotional concerns deemed this information more reliable and satisfying, a finding that was observed in both pro-vaccination and vaccine-hesitant groups. This study eloquently demonstrated that organizations should be mindful of the important differences in the manner information is provided to the public and attempts to correct misinformation online should be transparent and responsive to emotional aspects that patients and the public experience. In other words, "official" or professional organizations who use their social media platforms to sound "official" will likely have their messages, including those containing important evidence-based information, fall on deaf ears.

Lastly, as a testament to the rise of social media use among medical professionals, the number of peer-reviewed publications written for professionals as the target audience has also grown over the past few years. Multiple different specialties have published original articles, editorials, and "how to" guides for their readers. Some of these articles have addressed the basics of social media for beginners, others have focused on rationale for why medical professionals should join social media, and many have included guidance regarding best practices and professionalism. As we conclude this textbook, which was written for that exact purpose, we anticipate and collectively hope this trend will continue and will undoubtedly see additional textbooks and resources for medical professionals to use in their quest to develop their online personas and platforms.

This section on research offered a brief introduction into the types of articles being published in this realm. For those medical professionals engaged in academia and research of their own, this may offer inspiration for new areas of inquiry and opportunities for publication. For those who prefer to read and not write peer-reviewed articles, this may offer evidence of the growing use of social media among medical professionals, the acceptance by traditional medical journals (and essentially their governing professional organizations), and the type of data being analyzed to better understand these practices. Given the relative novelty of medical professionals using social media, there are countless opportunities for additional research and evaluation of the dissemination, efficacy, and even return on investment associated with these pursuits.

ZDoggMD

In this last section of our textbook, we would like to highlight the career of Zubin Damania, MD, who is better known as his online persona, ZDoggMD. There are multiple examples of well spoken, intelligent, and dedicated medical professionals who have used social media to reach a wide audience. Chapters 7 and 8 highlighted a few of these outstanding individuals, including Wendy Sue Swanson (SeattleMamaDoc), Eric Topol, and Kevin Pho (KevinMD). However, ZDoggMD is unparalleled in his approach to using social media to disseminate health-related information and is worthy of his own fun and educational case study.

Zubin Damania, MD, grew up in California and had two physician parents, both of whom emigrated from India (and serve as inspiration for some of his material). Dr. Damania received his undergraduate degree at University of California, Berkeley, and graduated from the University of California, San Francisco Medical School. Dr. Damania has an engaging and outgoing personality and an innate love of music and comedy. Early in his medical training, he began exploring the use of comedy to deliver medical information and developed stand-up comedy routines for medical organizations, pharmaceutical companies, and websites. He was one of two students invited to deliver a commencement speech at his own graduation from medical school, which was listed by National Public Radio as a top commencement speech of all time and has been viewed almost 150,000 times on YouTube [20].

Dr. Damania completed his residency training in internal medicine at Stanford University and worked as a hospitalist in Palo Alto for 10 years. Throughout this time, he continued his interesting side bar into comedy and became well known as a keynote presenter at medical conferences. Using his frustration for the traditional fee for service model that drove the American medical system *and* physician burnout as his muse, Dr. Damania started performing and filming musical parodies about all the frustrating aspects of being a physician and navigating the American medical system. This is when ZDoggMD was born (Fig. 11.2).

As ZDoggMD, Dr. Damania grew his social media presence and developed a worldwide audience. In addition to posting his musical parodies on YouTube, ZDoggMD has his own website and is very active on Facebook, Twitter, and Instagram. In the midst of developing his ZDoggMD persona and after 10 years as

Fig. 11.2 ZDoggMD in one of his musical parodies. (Used with permission from https://zdoggmd.com)

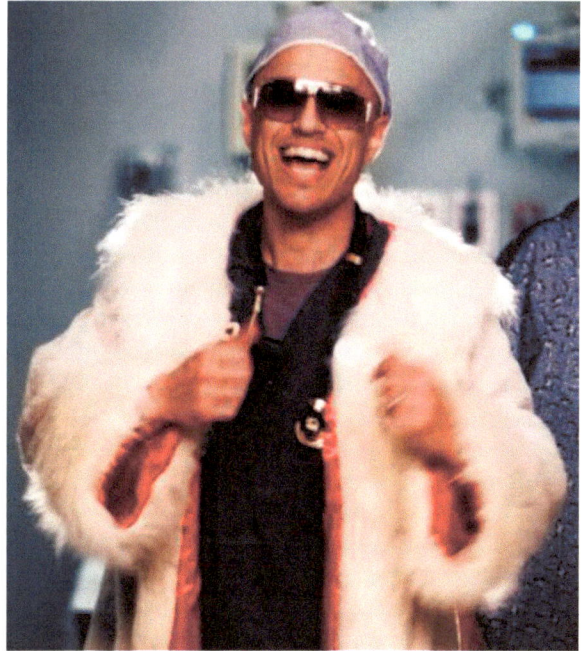

a practicing hospitalist (where he was honored for his dedication and outstanding teaching skills), Dr. Damania left his role as a hospitalist to found Turntable Health, a direct primary care clinic in downtown Las Vegas. In 2014, Dr. Damania announced his desire to lead a revolution titled "Healthcare 3.0," the goal of which is to revolutionize healthcare to return to personalized relationship-centered care that generates meaningful outcomes and removes the obsession with checking the boxes of administrative mandates and time wasting clicking of boxes in electronic medical records. ZDoggMD has been recognized by major media outlets as a healthcare influencer and continues to be a highly sought after keynote speaker at medical conferences across various specialties. ZDoggMD has expanded his social media pursuits and has developed a massive following on Facebook, accumulating almost two million followers. In 2017, ZDoggMD dedicated more time to his already popular Facebook show titled "Incident Report" and also launched an audio version of his Facebook Live recordings available via podcast.

ZDoggMD is much more than a physician who also happens to be an entertaining rapper and musical artist. He uses his significant platform to disseminate evidence-based health information on a wide variety of topics. He also prominently speaks out against the anti-vaccine movement, pseudoscience, violence in the health-related workplace, burnout, and issues pertaining to our less-than-ideal medical system, such as electronic medical records. ZDoggMD has interviewed prominent researchers and physicians on his popular podcast, which lends even more credibility to his information. Through a mixture of brutal honesty, comedy, memorable characters (Doc Vader is particularly humorous), musical genius, and a never ending lack of fear in trying new ideas, ZDoggMD has developed a massive and heterogenous audience consisting of medical trainees, nurses, physicians, healthcare administrators, media, and the general public. ZDoggMD endearingly refers to his followers as his "Tribe" and "ZPac." The last portion of the mission statement placed on his website says it all "The goal of our movement is to rapidly catalyze transformation by leveraging the awesome power of our passionate, engaged tribe of healthcare professionals. Join the ZPac and help us reclaim our calling!".

While most of us lack the amount of extroversion, talent, and internal drive that Zubin Damania possesses, his story can inspire us all to use social media to unleash our inner creativity and augment our desire to help others. As ZDoggMD demonstrates, there are no limits to the reach and approach medical professionals can utilize to disseminate evidence-based information and help countless individuals through social media.

Conclusion

If you have read this far, you have already demonstrated a desire to use your expertise to help others through social media. If you have read this entire book, you have already demonstrated that you are willing to take a different and necessary approach to using your expertise to help others. Even if, after reading this far, you still have no desire to join social media, at least you have gained an understanding of how our relationship with patients has already changed dramatically and will continue to do so moving forward. Regardless of what comes after you stop reading these pages, the editors and authors thank you for taking time out of your busy personal and professional lives to read our thoughts and consider our propositions. The best part about reading a textbook such as this is that you not only know where to find the authors but can reach them any time with questions or concerns. We hope you take advantage of that opportunity.

References

1. Dzau VJ, Ackerly DC, Sutton-Wallace P, Merson MH, Williams RS, Krishnan KR, Taber RC, Califf RM. The role of academic health science systems in the transformation of medicine. Lancet. 2010;375(9718):949–53.
2. Cabrera D, Vartabedian BS, Spinner RJ, Jordan BL, Aase LA, Timimi FK. More than likes and tweets: Creating social media portfolios for academic promotion and tenure. J Grad Med Educ. 2017;9(4):421–5.
3. Stukus DR. How I used Twitter to get promoted in academic medicine. KevinMD.com. 9 Oct 2016. https://www.kevinmd.com/blog/2016/10/used-twitter-get-promoted-academic-medicine.html. Last accessed: 4 Jan 2019.
4. Cabrera D, Roy D, Chisolm MS. Social media scholarship and alternative metrics for academic promotion and tenure. J Am Coll Radiol. 2018;15(1):135–41.
5. Chan TM, Stukus D, Leppink J, Duque L, Bigham BL, Mehta N, Thoma B. Social media and the 21st-century scholar: how you can harness social media to amplify your career. J Am Coll Radiol. 2018;15(1 Pt B):142–8.
6. Glassick CE. Boyer's expanded definitions of scholarship, the standards for assessing scholarship, and the elusiveness of the scholarship of teaching. Acad Med. 2000;75(9):877–80.
7. George DR, Rovniak LS, Kraschnewski JL. Dangers and opportunities for social media in medicine. Clin Obstet Gynecol. 2013;56(3):453–62.
8. Househ M. The use of social media in healthcare: organizational, clinical, and patient perspectives. Stud Health Technol Inform. 2013;183:244–8.
9. Ventola CL. Social media and health care professionals: benefits, risks, and best practices. P T. 2014;39(7):491–9.
10. Capurro D, Cole K, Echavarria MI, Joe J, Neogi T, Turner AM. The use of social networking sites for public health practice and research: a systematic review. J Med Internet Res. 2014;16(3):e79.
11. Zhang Z, Ahmed W. A comparison of information sharing behaviours across 379 health conditions on Twitter. Int J Public Health. 2018;64(3):431–40.
12. Carter M. Medicine and the media: how Twitter may have helped Nigeria contain Ebola. Br Med J. 2014;349:g6946.
13. Rosenzweig D, Nickels AS. #Asthma #Inhaler: evaluation of visual social media depictions of inhalers and spacers. J Allergy Clin Immunol Pract. 2017;5(6):1787–8.
14. Smailhodzic E, Hooijsma W, Boonstra A, Langley DJ. Social media use in healthcare: a systematic review of effects on patients and on their relationship with healthcare professionals. BMC Health Serv Res. 2016;16:442.
15. Soreide K, Mackenzie G, Polom K, Lorenzon L, Mohan H, Mayoi J. Tweeting the meeting: Quantitative and qualitative twitter activity during the 38th ESSO conference. Eur J Surg Oncol. 2019;45(2):284–9.
16. Wilkinson SE, Basto MY, Perovic G, Lawrentschuk N, Murphy DG. The social media revolution is changing the conference experience: analytics and trends from eight international meetings. BJU Int. 2015;115(5):639–46.

17. Alvarez-Perea A, Ojeda P, Zubeldia JM. Trends in Twitter use during the annual meeting of the Spanish Society of Allergology and Clinical Immunology (2013-2016). J Allergy Clin Immunol Pract. 2018;6(1):310–2.
18. Pemmaraju N, Thompson MA, Mesa RA, Desai T. Analysis of the use and impact of Twitter during American Society of Clinical Oncology Annual Meetings from 2011 to 2016: focus on advanced metrics and user trends. J Oncol Pract. 2017;13(7):e623–31.
19. Gesser-Edelsburg A, Diamant A, Hijazi R, Mesch GS. Correcting misinformation by health organizations during measles outbreaks: a controlled experiment. PLoS One. 2018;13(12):e0209505.
20. Funny graduation speech, UCSF Med School, ZDoggMD.com. https://www.youtube.com/watch?v=mgnHH7Iz37c. Last accessed 5 Jan 2019.

Index

A
Affect heuristic, 77
Aggregate bias, 74
Alzheimer's disease, 130, 141
Ambiguity effect, 75
America Online (AOL), 31, 32
Anchor, 77, 162
Anecdotes
    Dunning-Kruger effect, 69
    evidence-based resources, 67
    healthcare professionals, 69
    health literacy, 68
    medical information, 68
    patient privacy, 66, 67
    scientific method, 67, 68
Animoto, 163
Anti-vaccine sentiments, 6
Apple's Macintosh Operating System
        (Mac OS), 28
ARPANET, 24–27, 39
Asymmetric digital subscription line
        (ADSL), 33, 34
Audioblogging, 38
Availability heuristic, 77

B
BackRub, 36
Bad experience troll, 192, 193
Bandwagon effect, 75
Base-rate neglect, 75
Belief bias, 75
Blog posts, 151, 152
Blogs, 37
Broadband connections, 33, 34
Buzzsprout, 156
BuzzSumo, 160

C
Canva, 160, 163
Career development
    academic accomplishments, 205
    academic institutions, 204
    achievements, 204
    altmetrics, 204
    Assistant to Associate Professor of
            Pediatrics, 205
    digital and social media scholarship, 204
    guidelines, 204
    manuscript, 204
    objectives and platforms, 205
    peer-reviewed publications, 203, 204
    promotion and tenure committees, 204
    public health
        Centers for Disease Control, 206
        influenza activity, 206
        location tracking technology, 206
        natural disasters, 206
        organ-donor status, 206
        socioeconomic status, 206
        state and local health departments, 205
    research
        asthma, 207, 208
        conference hashtag, 209
        Ebola outbreak, 207
        evaluation of, 210
        health conditions, 207
        longitudinal analysis, 209
        number of publications, 206, 207
        online personas and platforms, 210
        patient-provider relationship, 208
        public encounter online, 207
        randomized controlled trial, 209, 210
        target audience, 207
        Twitter users, 206

© Springer Nature Switzerland AG 2019   215
D. R. Stukus et al., *Social Media for Medical Professionals*,
https://doi.org/10.1007/978-3-030-14439-5

Career development (*cont.*)
    types of articles, 210
    user's engagement, 209
    time lag prior, 204
    Twitter/Facebook, 204
    ZDoggMD
        American medical system, 211
        direct primary care clinic, 212
        electronic medical records, 212
        entertaining rapper and musical
            artist, 212
        examples, 210
        Facebook Live recordings, 212
        inner creativity and augment, 212
        media outlets, 212
        medical organizations, 211
        medical training, 211
        pharmaceutical companies, 211
        residency training, 211
        websites, 211
Cedars-Sinai Blog, 152
Classmates.com, 39
Classmates Online, 39
Cluster of European Research
        Projects (CERP), 28
Cognitive biases
    aggregate bias, 74
    ambiguity effect, 75
    bandwagon effect, 75
    base-rate neglect, 75
    belief bias, 75
    confirmation bias, 75
    framing effect, 75
    Hawthorne effect, 75
    illusory correlation, 75
    information bias, 75
    omission bias, 76
    online behavior, 74
    overconfidence bias, 76
    self-serving bias, 76
    YouGov, 74
Communication skills, 68
Community guidelines, 183
Complaint protocol, 183, 184
CompuServe, 25, 26, 31, 34
Computer Science Network (CSNET), 27
Conducting business, 182
Confidentiality
    data source availability, 175, 176
    de-identification, 174, 177
    distinguishability, 175, 176
    PHI, 174, 175
    replicability, 175, 176
    risk assessment, 175, 176

    social media usage, 175, 176
Confirmation bias, 74, 75
Content calendar, 149, 150
Content creation
    analyzing social media statistics, 168–170
    audience, 149
    content calendar, 149, 150
    content plan, 148, 149
    cross-post, 160, 161
    cross-promotion, 160
    edit your work, 166
    emotional appeal check, 166
    good content creation, 157–160
    good *vs.* great content, 166–168
    HIPAA and state privacy laws, 165
    original content, 146
    own content, 147, 148
    platforms for
        blog posts, 151, 152
        Facebook, 153
        Instagram, 156
        LinkedIn, 154
        Twitter, 154
        website, 151
        YouTube, 154, 155
    role models
        Dr. Howard Luks, 164
        Dr. Sandra Lee, 164
        Dr. Wendy Sue Swanson, 164–165
        New York Dynamic Neuromuscular
            Rehabilitation, 164
    rule of thumb, 165
    SEO factor, 146, 147
    tools
        Anchor, 162
        Animoto, 163
        Canva, 163
        Giphy, 162
        Grammarly, 162
        Hashtagify.me, 161
        Hootsuite, 163
        Placeit, 163
        Slideshare, 161
        SlideSnack, 162
        SurveyMonkey, 162
        Typeform, 163
        Typorama, 163
        Vidyard, 162
    violate patient privacy, 165
Content curation
    Alzheimer's care, 130
    amazing ideas, 140–142
    credibility online, 125, 126
    credibility red flags, 126, 127

Dr. Dave Stukus, 137, 138
Dr. Kevin Pho, 136, 137
Dr. Topol, Eric, 138, 139
encyclopedias, 121
Facebook, 121
finding credible sources, 124, 125
healthcare professionals on social media,
      127, 128
misuse of social media, 122
overarching theme, 130
private social media profiles, 131
promote health behaviors, 121
social media, 122, 123
      healthcare professionals, 128, 129
      helps patients, 129, 130
Step by Step Pediatrics, 132–134
Wendy Sue Swanson MD, 134–136
Creative Commons, 178
Creative Commons licenses, 178
Crisis communication, 184, 185
Cross promotion, 160
Cross-post, 160, 161
Curating content, 55
Cyborgs, 9

D
Daily Source Code, 38, 39
Damania, Zubin, 210–212
Data source availability, 175
Defamation, 180
De-identification, 174, 177
Democrat-backed policy, 191
Department of Defense, 23, 24, 27
Digital communications
      advanced browser and rise of websites,
            29–31
      America Online, 31, 32
      blogs, 37
      broadband connections, 33, 34
      Compu-Serv, 25
      internet, 28, 29
      network growth, 27
      Physicians Online (POL), 32
      podcasts, 38–39
      RSS feeds, 38
      search engines, 35
            BackRub, 36
            Google, 36
            JumpStation, 35
            WebCrawler, 35
            Yahoo, 35
      smartphones and mobile apps, 42–44
      social networking sites, 39–42

Classmates Online, 39
development, 42
Facebook, 40, 41
Friendster, 40
LinkedIn, 40
MySpace, 40
SixDegrees, 40
Twitter, 41, 42
usenet and newsgroups, 25, 26
web programming languages, 36, 37
WorldWideWeb, 28, 29
Distinguishability, 175, 176
Doximity, 20
Dunning-Kruger effect, 69

E
Echo chamber effect, 73, 74
Endorsements, 181
ePocrates, 31
Evidence-based medicine, 54, 68
Evidence-based resources, 67
Explicit content, 180, 181
Extremist troll, 195, 196

F
Facebook, 2, 5, 10–12, 20, 40, 41, 50, 121,
      122, 129, 132–135, 153, 155, 156
      features, 11
      for healthcare professionals, 12
      Instant Articles program, 11
      issues, 11
      Nationwide Children's Hospital,
            homepage for, 11
      News Feed, 10
      tag feature, 11
      Timeline, 10
FaceMash, 40, 41
Fair use, 176, 178
False statements, 179
File transfer protocol (FTP), 24
Firefox, 30
Framing effect, 75
Friendster, 40

G
GameLine, 31
General Electric's GEnie Network, 25
Giphy, 162
Google, 20, 30, 36, 43, 71, 86, 93, 94, 99, 109,
      124, 136, 146, 147
Google Alerts, 71, 140, 157

Google Analytics, 169
Google Maps, 145
Google Scholar, 86, 203
Grammar and Spelling Troll, 190
Grammarly, 162
Great content, 166

H
Harassment, 180, 190, 195, 196
Hashtagify.me, 161
Hashtags, 16, 17
Hawthorne effect, 75
Healthcare consumers, 52–53
Healthcare Finance, 49
Healthcare professionals, 68, 69
    anecdotes, 69
    evidence-based information
        and interactions, 80
    iconic paintings and lasting images, 80
    limitations, 80
    medical advice, 81
    personal advice, 81, 82
    professional organizations and academic
        hospital systems, 80
    responsibility, 80
    visibility and accessibility, 81
Health Insurance Portability and
    Accountability Act of 1996
    (HIPAA), 58, 174, 179,
    183, 192
Health literacy, 68
Heuristic technique
    affect heuristic, 77
    anchoring, 77
    availability, 77
    development, 76
    escalation of commitment, 77
    representativeness, 77
Hootsuite, 55, 117, 163
Human nature, 66
Hypertext transfer protocol (http), 27

I
Illusory correlation, 75
Infection, 5, 65, 66, 109, 132
Influenza vaccine, 6, 65, 66
Information bias, 75
Instagram, 2, 14–16, 156
Insult troll, 192
Integrated Digital Services Network
    (ISDN), 33, 36
Intellectual property, 176, 178

Interface Message Processor (IMP), 24
Internet, 2, 28, 29
Internet Explorer, 29
Internet Manager's Phonebook, 28
Internet trolls
    anonymity, 197
    bad experience troll, 192, 193
    definition, 189
    extremist troll, 195, 196
    grammar and spelling troll, 190
    harassment, 190
    healthy and productive debate online,
        198, 200
    herd mentality, 197
    insult troll, 192
    options, 196
    personality, 197
    Political Troll, 190–192
    topic troll, 193–195
    vaccinations and circumcision, 197
iPodder, 39
ISDN, *see* Integrated Digital Services
    Network (ISDN)
iTunes, 55, 156

L
Libsyn, 156
LinkedIn, 20, 40, 154, 156

M
Macromedia Flash, 36
Mayo Clinic, 123
Mayo Clinic Academic Appointments and
    Promotions Committee, 204
Media relations, 182, 183
Medical information, 68
Medline, 31
MedlinePlus, 123
Medscape, 31
Mozilla Foundation, 30
MySpace, 40, 50

N
Napster, 38, 40
National Information Infrastructure
    Protection Act, 33
National Science Foundation Network
    (NSFNET), 27–29
NCSA Mosaic, 29
Newsreaders, 26
Non-evidence based medicine, 69

O

Omission bias, 76
2016 Online Harassment
 Study, 190
Open Diary, 37
Organizational reputation, 186
Organizational use, 173
Overconfidence bias, 76

P

PageRank, 36
Palm Operating System, 43
Palm Pilot, 42, 43
Patient privacy, 66, 67
PediaCast, 39, 155
Personal digital assistant (PDA),
 42, 43
Photos and videos, 179
Physicians Online (POL), 32
Pinterest, 5, 19, 20
Placeit, 163
Podbean, 156
Podcasts, 38–39
Podsafe Music Network, 39
Political troll, 190–192
Private Health Information (PHI),
 174, 175
Prodigy, 25, 34
Productive debate online, 198, 200
Professional boundaries, 185, 186
Pseudoscience 101
 chronic conditions, 78
 definition, 77
 Dunning-Kruger effect, 78
 evidence-based information, 78
 medical information, 79
 qualifications, 78
 website, 79
 words and phrases, 78, 79
PubMed, 86, 106, 108, 109, 203, 207

Q

Quality evidence
 clinical guideline, 70
 cognitive biases and pseudoscience, 70
 headlines media outlets, 71
 media reports, 71, 72
 misinterpretation, 71
 online discussions, 71
 scientific evidence, 70
 Twitter, 71
Quantum Link, 31

R

Reddit, 19, 94, 96
Replicability, 175
Representativeness heuristic, 77
Republican-backed policy, 191
Rich Site Summary (RSS) feeds, 38
Risk assessment, 175
Road Runner High Speed Online, 34

S

Safe Harbor method, 174
Scientific method, 67, 68
Search Engine Watch, 49
Search engines, 35, 37
 BackRub, 36
 Google, 36
 JumpStation, 35
 WebCrawler, 35
 Yahoo, 35
Self-serving bias, 76
SixDegrees, 40
Slideshare, 161
SlideSnack, 162
Snapchat, 19, 50, 51, 175, 181
Social media, 55, 56
 benefits of, 60, 61
 bots and rise of fake news, 8, 9
 curating content, 55
 cyberbullying, 4
 definition of, 1, 4
 Doximity, 20
 education and recommendations
  online motivates, 61
 evidence-based medicine, 54
 evidence-based recommendations
  and guidelines, 53
 Facebook, 10–12
 free open-access medical education, 60
 Going viral, 5
 Google, 20
 health and wellness, 49–50
 healthcare consumers, 52–53
 healthcare decisions, 53
 Instagram, 14–16
 interactive applications, 1
 LinkedIn, 20
 medical outcomes, 53
 millennials, 50, 51
  age, percentage of Americans, 51
  older Americans, 51
  sex, education and income, 51
 misconceptions, 54, 61
 opinion-rendering translates, 57

Social media (*cont.*)
  opportunities, 60
  out with the old, 2–3
  patient-provider relationship, 59
  Pinterest, 19, 20
  policy, 173, 174
  to political opinions, 53
  practical steps for medical professionals, 62
  professional liability, 54
  profiles, 1
  Reddit, 19
  risks, 58, 59
  signs of, 3
  smartphone, 3
  Snapchat, 19
  social networks, 2, 10
  time commitment, 54
  Twitter, 5, 6, 8, 16–18
  types of, 4
  user generated content, 1
  viral tweets, 6–8
  YouTube, 12–14
Social networking sites, 39–42
  Classmates Online, 39
  development, 42
  Facebook, 40, 41
  Friendster, 40
  LinkedIn, 40
  MySpace, 40
  SixDegrees, 40
  Twitter, 41, 42
SoundCloud, 156
Student Doctor Network, 31
SurveyMonkey, 162, 163

T
T-1 backbone, 27
Threats, 179
Timeline, 10
Topic troll, 193–195
Transmission Control Protocol/Internet
      Protocol (TCP/IP), 24
Twitter, 2, 5, 6, 8, 16–18, 41, 121, 122, 125,
      126, 129, 132, 134, 136–140, 154,
      156, 198
  accounts/individuals questions, 105
  allergic and immunologic conditions, 102
  audience engagement and interest
      account analytics, 117, 118
      data collection and sharing, 120
      examples, 118
      positive feedback and reinforcement, 119
      terminology, 119

Choosing Wisely campaign, 109
clinical setting, 107
content curation and creation, 105
content sharing, 105
Cyber bullying, 17
elevator speech, 102
emotional/argumentative reply, 111
evidence and clinical guidelines, 107
evidence-based medicine, 101
Facebook groups, 109, 110
features, 110, 111
gifs, 17
Google, 109
hashtags, 16, 102, 105
  examples, 115
  inappropriate content, 115
  index keywords/topics, 114
  live Twitter chats, 116
  medical conferences, 115
  meeting hashtag, 115
  networking, 116
  spaces, symbols/punctuation, 114
  subtle differences, 115
healthcare, examples of, 101
for healthcare professionals, 18
home page, 102
individual accounts, 102
intellectual journey, 105
interests, professional affiliations,
      and links, 103
interpretation of statistics, 108
journal articles, 106
media reports, 106
medical accounts, 102
medical conferences, 106
medical recommendations, 109
medications, 108
micro blogging, 110
minded medical professional, 105
new followers, 104
non-medical professionals, 108
online dialogue, 106
online reputation, 111
patient perspective, 108, 109
patient privacy, 106, 107
patients, colleagues, and media, 107
peer reviewed journals, 108
personal experiences, 106
practice of medicine, 108
principles, 111
professional/personal
      purposes, 101
professional portrait, 102, 103
professionalism standards, 102

publications, education, and
    background, 103
PubMed, 109
quality information, 104
questions/comments, 111
real-life clinical encounters, 106
research methodology, 108
retweeting, 16
scientific method, 108
search engine algorithms, 108
sharing of opinions and emotional
    responses, 16
target audience, 104
time management, 116, 117
trending topics, 105
    adult references, 112
    algorithm, 111
    breaking news, 111
    celebrities/popular sporting events, 111
    discrimination, 112
    inappropriate content, 111
    by location, 112
    non-medical trending topics, 113
    personal presence, 112
    popular media stories, 111
    professional presence, 112
    search results, 112
    settings feature, 112
    tragic events, 112
tweet, 16
Twitter handles, 101
users, 101
value for audience, 105
Vartabedian, Bryan, 104

Typeform, 163, 168
Typorama, 159, 163

U
Uniform Resource Locator (URL), 28

V
Vaccine Adverse Event Reporting
    System (VAERS), 52
Vaccines, 6, 54, 55, 66, 84, 148, 194
Vidyard, 162

W
Web programming languages, 36, 37
WebCrawler, 35
Weblog, 37
WebMD, 30, 32, 123
Website, 151
Wired Magazine, 125
World Wide Web, 28, 29, 35, 37, 39

Y
Yahoo, 35, 36
YouTube, 12–14, 154, 155
    face-to-face interaction, 13
    growing aspect of, 13
    for healthcare professionals, 13, 14
    motivated users, 12
    negative aspects, 13
    sharing entertainment/information, 12